The M&M Files

Morbidity and Mortality
Rounds in
Emergency Medicine

The M&M Files

Morbidity and Mortality Rounds in Emergency Medicine

Frank J. Edwards, MD, FACEP

Clinical Associate Professor of Emergency Medicine
University of Rochester Medical Center
Rochester, NY

President
Delphi Emergency Physician Services, LLC
Williamson, NY

HANLEY & BELFUS, INC. / Philadelphia

Publisher: HANLEY & BELFUS, INC.
                  Medical Publishers
                  210 South 13th Street
                  Philadelphia, PA 19107
                  (215) 546-7293; 800-962-1892
                  FAX (215) 790-9330
                  Web site: http://www.hanleyandbelfus.com

Disclaimer: Although the information in this book has been carefully reviewed for correctness of dosage and indications, neither the authors nor the editor nor the publisher can accept any legal responsibility for any errors or omissions that may be made. Neither the publisher nor the editor makes any warranty, expressed or implied, with respect to the material contained herein. Before prescribing any drug, the reader must review the manufacturer's current production information (package inserts) for accepted indications, absolute dosage recommendations, and other information pertinent to the safe and effective use of the product described.

Library of Congress Control Number: 2002104832

M&M Files
Morbidity and Mortality Rounds in Emergency Medicine   ISBN 1-56053-540-7

Last digit is the print number: 9 8 7 6 5 4 3 2 1

Dedication

This book is dedicated to the physicians I work with; to Mary Ann (my constant source of inspiration); to its fine editor, Kathleen Kolsun, MD; and to all our patients.

CONTENTS

Introduction and Risk Management

Every other month after the emergency department staff meeting, we clear the room of nonphysicians, fill our coffee cups, close the door, and present all of the cases that have generated negative outcomes or complaints since the last meeting. Sometimes the physician presents his or her own case, but many of the cases we leave anonymous. The point, after all, is to learn from the experience of others, not to embarrass anyone. Physicians with cases on the list already have had the issue hashed out to whatever degree was necessary. But an interesting thing happens. Frequently a person will drop by later and ask if this or that anonymous case belonged to him or her, even though physicians should know that a case is never sprung on them unannounced at a group meeting. The physician had empathized so completely with the situation that it became indistinguishable from his or her own experience.

This telling phenomenon touches on two important points about morbidity and mortality (M&M) rounds. First, we all share a great number of common clinical dilemmas. Secondly, case presentations can engage us emotionally as well as intellectually. It is a fact of life that some cases have bad outcomes, and no one gets it perfect every time. Most physicians possess—in fact, need to possess—a healthy fear of harming patients. During an M&M presentation, this fear rises close to the surface as we become vicariously riveted to the details, imagining how we would have handled the case, wondering if we would have stumbled into the same pitfalls. M&M rounds, therefore, can be as educational as real life, even bearing some of the same emotional distress.

For emergency department medical directors concerned about minimizing their department's rate of complaints and adverse outcomes, M&M rounds are part of the feedback process whereby the entire group receives a fine-tuning of clinical judgment and knowledge base.

This book includes cases gathered from M&M rounds from a number of sources. Because a good M&M session takes a fair amount of time and is usually restricted to cases within a given institution, this book hopes to supplement the M&M Rounds in both teaching and community hospitals, allowing program directors and medical directors to expose trainees and colleagues to a greater range and number of cases than otherwise might be possible.

Case-based learning is effective because interesting "stories" peak our attention and place facts in context. Along with considerations of diversity, the cases in this book were selected for qualities of interest. Details have been changed when necessary to protect patient confidentiality. M&M rounds, if you'll forgive a military metaphor, resemble a platoon of men and women huddled at the edge of a forest as one of their number strides forth into a mine field. If the life of an emergency physician is full of daily mine field excursions, the role of the medical director is to mark the correct path and pick up the pieces. And that is what an M&M session does.

During a good M&M conference, time flies, new ideas arise, confessions are made, vulnerability and frustrations are expressed, and a greater sense of community and purpose arises. In short, it can provide inspiration and catharsis. Beyond that, we should let the cases speak for themselves.

But first, some thoughts about risk management. Several years ago I had the privilege of writing a book about medical malpractice. I wanted to see which of the many arguments about the "malpractice crisis" were true and to what extent. Was it a matter of too many bad doctors protecting each other? Was it the fault of greedy malpractice attorneys taking advantage of the contingency fee system? Was it just an aspect of an overly litigious society? I studied both historical and current statistics and looked in depth at a number of malpractice cases. Not surprisingly, every argument contained its own slice of validity, and the conclusions of the book were less than earth-shattering.

But out of that research, I discovered an interesting paradigm that has helped me over the years. Every time a physician enters into a relationship with a patient, four distinct and separate scales arise—four variables that separate a good case from a bad case:

1. The first factor is simply the severity of the disease process. How bad is the illness? How much potential does it have for causing harm? On the left side of this curve lie problems such as minor sprains and runny noses. On the right lie the subarachnoid hemorrhage and multisystem trauma.

2. The second factor is the obscurity with which the disease presents. Some clinical problems present exactly as the textbooks describe them; others are barely recognizable from the clinical

clues. An acute myocardial infarction may present in classic textbook fashion or like a case of temporomandibular joint syndrome. An atrial myxoma may be found incidentally on a routine echocardiogram or present with vague, intermittent spells, in which the patient complains, "My head feels funny."

3. The third factor is the provider's astuteness during a particular encounter. A physician's diagnostic acumen is founded on his or her native talent in combination with experience and training but varies significantly depending on fatigue, distractions, underlying emotional states, physical health, and so forth.

4. The fourth factor is the quality of the physician-patient interaction. In most cases, a reasonable degree of mutual respect and warmth quickly develops between doctor and patient. But there are always many negative emotions in the emergency department, even for physicians with a natural gift for winning the patient's confidence and respect—and some physicians cannot seem to help but leave a wake of animosity behind them.

Bad outcomes can be generated if any one of these factors is negative, but outcomes worsen in proportion to the total number of negative factors. The encounter becomes especially problematic when both factors one and two are negative. Consider a man who dies of a myocardial infarction in the emergency department following correct, timely diagnosis and treatment by a physician who developed a positive relationship with patient and family. There is little chance of a complaint, and certainly no lawsuit would be successful.

In general, all four factors must be negative to create a major problem or a significant lawsuit: a truly serious disease presenting in an obscure fashion to a physician who is not at his or her sharpest in the context of a less-than-ideal patient interaction. The consequences are almost guaranteed to be poor for everyone concerned.

Clearly, factors one and two are beyond the clinician's control. But factors three and four, problem-solving powers and rapport with patients, we can hone and fine-tune. An excellent way to accomplish this goal is by watching the four factors play out in real cases. If experience is the best teacher, then we and, in turn, our patients have much to gain by studying the experiences of our colleagues.

Frank J. Edwards, M.D., FACEP

Case 1
The Child from Hell

A two-and-a-half year old boy fell on the playground and was brought into the emergency department by his parents shortly after 6 PM, complaining of pain in his right arm. The triage nurse reported swelling around the wrist; the child was anxious and tearful. Because the department was extremely busy, the nurse obtained a verbal order for acetaminophen, which seemed to help the child feel better. But by 9:30 PM, when the child was finally brought to a room, the analgesic effect had worn off. The physician took a quick look at the arm and sent the patient for x-rays, with a warning to the x-ray techician that he was "the child from hell." The x-ray techician apparently agreed and informed the parents, as they helped restrain their son for radiographs, that he understood why the emergency physician had called the boy "the child from hell."

The emergency physician diagnosed a slightly angulated "green-stick" fracture of the radius and ulna. While applying a plaster splint, according to the parents, the physician ordered the nurse to hold the boy down, then he looked into his eyes and said, "You are the worst patient I've ever worked on."

The physician himself did not recall using those exact words, but the parents were quite specific. They reported that his comment did not make the child more cooperative.

After applying the splint, the emergency physician contacted the child's pediatrician to arrange follow-up, and during this conversation once again he used the phrase, "child from hell." At least that is what the pediatrician told the parents the next day when they visited her office.

The parents wrote an open letter to the hospital CEO and board of directors and sent a copy to the local newspaper. The well-written epistle described their long wait in the emergency department and the physician's attitude and comments. They stated that under no circumstances would they visit that department again; they would drive 50 miles in the opposite direction, if necessary. They would not take an animal there for treatment, let alone a child. The letter was published on the editorial page under the title, "Our Emergency Room Going to the Dogs."

Analysis

Patients and families frequently tolerate crowded conditions and long delays—as long as they feel that the caregivers treat them with respect and do their best. Respect is conveyed through tact. Negative comments by people outside the nuclear family about a child's behavior—in any setting—are usually not well received by parents. In this case, the combination of a long wait plus a few tactless comments triggered a public expression of discontent that damaged an emergency department's reputation.

Teaching Points

1. One of the best possible risk-management tools is empathy on the part of the physician.

2. Avoid the verbalization of judgmental comments that may be misconstrued as insults by patients or family.

Case 2
Hold that Cigarette

A 69-year-old man with terminal chronic obstructive pulmonary disease (COPD) came by ambulance late one night to the emergency department. His wife arrived by car a few minutes later. His shortness of breath had worsened throughout the day. The wife called the primary physician that afternoon and was told to increase his oxygen from 2 to 3 liters per minute. She was reluctant to do so because a neighbor had told her that too much oxygen is dangerous for a person with severe lung disease.

The man's oxygen saturation was 96% when he arrived at the emergency department. He was taking 50% oxygen by Venturi mask and was reasonably comfortable. His breath sounds were poor, however, and the emergency physician ordered a series of nebulized bronchodilator treatments as well as a dose of intravenous solumedrol to supplement chronic prednisone treatment. A chest x-ray showed no acute changes. Looking though the man's old chart, the emergency physician discovered that during an emergency department visit several weeks ago the social worker had begun planning for hospice care. After a few hours in the emergency department, the patient's oxygen saturation stabilized in the low nineties on 3 liters of oxygen per minute. Blood gas analysis was not significantly worse than previous studies, and the patient reported a return to his usual state of respiratory misery. The emergency physician reviewed the case by telephone with the primary care doctor, who agreed that it would be reasonable to send the patient home.

The patient's wife, however, seemed surprised. The emergency physician spent several minutes informing her that nothing more could be done, but she was not reassured. When he offered to call social services in the morning to facilitate the hospice process, she became almost hostile.

The emergency physician sent the patient home, but the primary physician admitted him to the hospital on the following day after repeated calls from the wife. During the admission, she demanded an audience with the hospital administrator. She told him that the emergency physician had acted rudely and inappropriately in discharging her husband from the emergency department. As an example of his callousness, she pointed to the fact that he had written on the discharge instructions for the patient to quit smoking. She felt that the instruction was just a "cruel joke" because it was too late to help.

The patient died several days later. The administrator received two more phone calls from the man's children, echoing their mother's anger at the emergency physician.

Analysis

A thorough review of the emergency department record clearly showed that the emergency physician's evaluation and treatment fell within good standards of care and that the decision to discharge was medically appropriate and in no way related to the patient's demise. How could the emergency physician have avoided these complaints, all of which found their way into his peer review file, and brought him center stage during an M&M conference?

This was an emotionally difficult time for the patient's wife, who was not yet ready to accept the inevitability of her husband's death. The emergency physician made an attempt to "educate" her, which was fine and good—if it had been done in an appropriately sensitive fashion. But denial is among the strongest forces in human consciousness. The emergency physician elected not to bow to it, however, and the interaction deteriorated into what the patient's wife perceived as an argument.

The emergency physician failed to recognize that he was treating two patients—the husband and his wife. Although he gave the husband good medicine, the wife received an unpalatable nostrum that only heightened her discomfort.

Sensitivity is the key. When faced with the wife's resistance, the emergency physician should have recognized immediately that he had entered a second realm, where the language is different and phrases such as "medical appropriateness" lack meaning. If he had switched gears and coasted into empathy with the patient's wife by dealing with her suffering on its own terms, in all likelihood he could have walked her through the situation, and both would have emerged unscathed. Such a relationship may be difficult to achieve in the emergency department setting. If the emergency physician encounters a situation in which he or she cannot resolve an issue, the primary physician may be brought into the loop. The patient's primary doctor was on duty that night. Nothing prevented the emergency physician from calling the primary doctor back and putting him on the phone with the wife to discuss options.

But that solution did not occur to the physician, and the patient's wife left angry and unsatisfied. The emergency physician's final gesture of medical appropriateness was the message on the discharge sheet, written in capitals with an exclamation point—QUIT SMOKING!

To what end? The advice that we give our patients must be practical and have a purpose, or it may spin out of control. Enough said.

Teaching Points

1. Emergency physicians must remain sensitive to the emotional state of the family and loved ones of patients. They, in essence, become "patients" as well.

2. Issues of terminal care must be dealt with delicately and in concert with primary physicians, whenever feasible.

3. Avoid comments on discharge instructions that may be perceived as derogatory or judgmental.

4. Medical appropriateness and good outcomes do not always go hand in hand. The emergency physician must not become "tone deaf" to emotional issues surrounding a case.

Case 3
The Vigorous Examiner

While walking down his front steps one winter morning, an elderly gentleman slipped on a patch of ice, striking the left side of his chest on a railing. He came to the emergency department and after a brief wait was ushered into a treatment room. The emergency physician briskly examined him, listening to and palpating his chest. "I was glad he came in right away," the man said in a later conversation with the medical director, "but he was really rough. He poked my chest so hard I had to yelp, and he kept on pushing. I felt like smacking the son-of-a-bitch." The emergency physician also palpated the man's abdomen. It was noted as being soft and nontender in all quadrants.

The emergency physician ordered a chest x-ray. When the man returned from radiology, the emergency physician read the films as negative and discharged the patient with a diagnosis of chest wall contusion and instructions to use ibuprofen if he had any pain. ("The pain was awful. I could hardly get a good breath. That 'iprobufferin' didn't help me at all.")

The following afternoon, the patient received a phone call from the emergency department. "They asked me first how I was doing—and oh, by the way, sir, the doctor seems to have overlooked two broken ribs." Shortly after this call, the patient telephoned the hospital president as well as the chairman of the board of trustees to complain of his rough treatment and the misdiagnosis.

Analysis

To empathize with the discomfort that patients may experience during an exam and to minimize such discomfort whenever possible is not only compassionate medicine but also lessens the chance that the patient will feel dissatisfied with his care. The physician certainly did not intend to cause the patient excessive pain; however, the patient walked away from the emergency department feeling distinctly worse than when he had entered—not to mention disgruntled by the physi-

6

cian's lack of empathy. Physicians behave in this manner at their medicolegal peril. If a complication had developed, can anyone doubt that a serious suit would have followed?

No one likes practicing in an environment of medicolegal fear, but we live in a society that nurtures the desire to seek redress and in which attorneys bend over backward to accommodate that desire. A malpractice suit represents the ultimate breakdown in rapport with a patient. If there was no rapport to begin with—as in this case—the chance of a suit multiplies.

The physician was in a rush to elicit a physical sign and did not commiserate with the patient's discomfort. It would have cost him a few seconds at best to prepare the patient with a simple statement—such as "This may hurt, but I need to check you out"—followed by recognition of the discomfort and an apology. A simple human connection would have been made and the pain of the exam forgiven.

Most emergency physicians at one time or another have missed a rib fracture, and in most cases such an oversight is no major problem. The real issue lies in the potential for complications. Some emergency physicians find it wise simply to tell any patient with chest trauma and apparently negative x-rays that they may have an occult rib fracture. If the radiologist sees something, the hospital will call the patient. Such comments would have added approximately 15 seconds to the physician–patient interaction, but they also would have satisfied the patient and aborted a complaint.

Establishing a good rapport with patients may be more difficult in the emergency department than in an office setting, but it is even more important. It simply involves recognizing the emotional dimension to every patient encounter and dealing with it as one friend to another.

Teaching Point

1. Always prepare a patient verbally for parts of an exam or procedure that may be painful.

2. If you inflict pain on a patient, an apology is always appropriate.

Case 4
The Body Unprepared

A 52-year-old man with a history of cardiac risk factors collapsed at home. The family began cardiopulmonary resuscitation. By the time the patient arrived in the emergency department, however, he had regained no cardiac activity. Resuscitation efforts proved equally futile, and the patient was pronounced dead in the emergency department.

The deceased man's brother called and wrote the hospital administration several days later. Although he said that the nurse and doctor who cared for her brother were "excellent," several aspects of the emergency department experience had caused the family great emotional pain. First, they felt "badgered" for insurance information by the registration clerk while resuscitation efforts were still under way. Second, and by far more disturbing, was the fact that when they went into the room to view the body after pronouncement, the endotracheal tube was still in place and the monitor was still attached, displaying a flat line.

Analysis

Our first response may be to discount this story, believing that the endotracheal tube was left in place pending release by the medical examiner. But investigation revealed that such was not the case. The medical examiner, in fact, was actually in the emergency department during the resuscitation efforts and had formally released the body. No autopsy was to be performed. Nonetheless, no one thought to remove the ET tube. It was still in place the next morning, when the funeral director picked up the body from the morgue. When the director told the family, they were even more upset.

Whether or not the ET tube was left in the patient's throat, it is clear that *no one prepared the family properly* for what they would see. The fact that the providers did not tell the family about the ET tube (confirmed by speaking with several family members) and that no one bothered to turn off the monitor clearly suggest a breakdown of protocol. Obviously everyone believed that someone else would take the responsibility to prepare the body for viewing by the family and to prepare the family for viewing the body.

The family requested a meeting with the ED director, which took place several months after the patient's death. The patient had been a popular, highly visible person in the community, and the several family members at the meeting were reasonable people. Their grief was still strongly in evidence, clearly exacerbated by how the patient's body had been treated. The only mollifying factor was the fact that they truly felt that the nurse and doctor had done a "wonderful job."

This resuscitation was unsuccessful from more than one standpoint. The treatment of a person who dies in the emergency department includes dealing with the emotional state of the survivors. This part of treatment is not optional—it is one of the most important aspects. If it is not handled properly, the emotional sequelae can be severe.

Ordinarily, someone—usually the nurse—takes responsibility for preparing the body and the family for viewing. The emergency physician is ultimately responsible for this procedure, however, and cannot simply assume that it will be done appropriately.

Teaching Points

1. Emergency departments should have a formal policy for the viewing of bodies by loved ones and family members.

2. The policy should outline the factors involved in optimal preparation for viewing, which should include, to whatever extent is reasonable, the wiping away of blood and vomitus from the face, the removal of tubes in orifices, and the placement of a clean sheet up to the patient's chin.

3. The policy should indicate who takes responsibility for this preparation.

4. A staff member—ideally the physician or the primary nurse— should accompany family members into a room for viewing of the body. The physician or nurse should prepare the family for anything out of the ordinary—such as disfiguring trauma or continued presence of endotracheal or nasogastric tubes and why they might be still be in place (e.g., awaiting evaluation by medical examiners).

5. Lastly, registration personnel must be sensitized to the fact that the procurement of insurance and demographic information from the family members of deceased patients may need to take a second seat to emotional priorities.

Case 5
A Fit of Pique

A young woman was carrying her 18-month-old daughter down a flight of steps at home. Near the bottom, her foot slipped and she fell. Although she managed to twist and avoid falling on the child, the child's head came into forceful contact with a heating grate. The baby began crying immediately. Her only visible injury was a cut to the forehead, which was bleeding profusely. The mother immediately drove to the emergency department, where she had an experience that generated the following letter of complaint [excerpted]:

> After we waited about an hour and a half in the room, Dr. X came in. He said to take the ice pack off because it wasn't doing any good, which was true because it had been on so long. Then he had the nurse strap Jessica into a papoose board so he could stitch her. He numbed up the cut and then proceeded to pick up an instrument from the tray to begin stitching. He abruptly threw down the instrument, and said very loudly "he couldn't work with this." He said it had to be thrown away, and then he ripped off his gloves and stomped out of the room while the nurse went somewhere to find another instrument. He seemed to be in a major huff. I saw him go across the hall and start looking at another patient who had come in long after we did. The nurse had to finally go get him. He finished stitching her, but I couldn't even talk, I was so appalled he would walk out like that with Jessica still in the papoose board crying. And I'm sure the way he acted made her even more frightened.

> I have worked as a nursing assistant for several years and feel that Dr. X's behavior was extremely unprofessional and rude. If the instruments are inadequate in the ER, then I urge the hospital to fix this problem, but I'm mainly writing to tell you about this and to say I do not think I will ever be comfortable coming to your ER again, no matter whether Dr. X is there or not, or whether he bothers to apologize, because I'm not sure I'd even want to hear it now.

Analysis

This case needs little further discussion. Although the child's laceration did well, a fact confirmed by the family's pediatrician in follow-up, the negative impression given by the emergency physician will always linger. Patients are not interested in our frustrations, nor should they be exposed to them. Any relief that the physician experienced by venting his anger was more than erased by the discomfort of having his behavior discussed in several forums, spending less-than-pleasant time across the desk from the CEO, and writing letters of apology.

If the outcome had been less than happy, the physician would have faced even more discomfort of a legal nature.

Teaching Points

1. Unprofessional behavior is frequently shocking to patients and will long be remembered, no matter how professional the care or how good the outcome.

2. Concerns about the adequacy of instruments or supplies in an emergency department should be taken directly to the medical director or nursing supervisor; they should not be mentioned in front of patients.

Case 6
Another Crier

The following letter reached the hospital CEO's desk via the billing office:

> I am returning this bill to you and let me tell you exactly why. My sister had brought me into the ER because I had been very depressed. I didn't really want to be there, but I didn't know where else to go and I needed some help. They put me into the room right across from the ER desk and I could hear everything going on. The doctor was standing there talking to someone on the phone. He was getting more and more angry. He was almost yelling about something I think a nurse had done, but I don't know for sure. He hung up the phone and walked into the room with me. He sat down in the chair and asked me two questions. He said "are you hurting anywhere?" I told him no. Then he asked me "are you thinking of hurting yourself?" I couldn't answer because I started crying, which was one of the problems that brought me in to begin with. He got up abruptly and said to a nurse out in the hallway, "another crier." About half an hour later, the psychiatry nurse came in and I ended up being sent out to see a counselor.
>
> The point is that because of the way Dr. Y treated me—the unprofessional way he acted on the phone in front of me, and then what he said in the hallway—I left your ER feeling humiliated and worse than when I came in. I cannot justify paying Dr. Y any type of fee for the less than one minute of time he spent with me, and the way he said "another crier." How can you possibly expect payment for this kind of treatment?

Analysis

Emergency department directors sometimes express the thought that emergency physicians tend to fall into two groups: (1) good *technical* doctors and (2) good *people* doctors. Technical doctors possess great proficiency with airway control measures and surgical procedures. They love to drop transvenous pacemakers, pop in chest tubes, and hang propofol drips. People doctors, on the other hand, have a gift for empathizing with another person's psychic condition and enhancing the overall emotional microclimate of an interaction. In short, they like patients and are well liked in return. The ideal emergency physician, obviously, excels in both realms.

The emergency doctor involved in the case described above was a renowned "techie," widely viewed by the entire staff to be the doctor whom they would want on duty if they came in after an accident or an acute myocardial infarction. But a complaint like this suggests an almost malicious, if not reckless, disregard for the patient's emotional state. Granted, her life was not at risk . . . but was it?

Rudeness is completely preventable. Rudeness creates a barrier of animosity, which, no matter how subtle, can impede the flow of critical information that a physician needs to take appropriate steps. Physicians who do not believe that compassion is a necessary good unto itself can at least view it as a tool to make communication more productive and prevent the nuisance and embarrassment of complaints. The key is empathy, which simply means achieving a nonjudgmental understanding of the patient's point of view. Do not say or do anything to a patient that you yourself would not find acceptable if the shoe were on the other foot. Most good physicians recognize that when they are at the bedside their function is, to a degree, theatrical. Tens of thousands of times they will be asked to play the "role" of the healer, and they must act the part, which means relegating personal prejudices, frustrations, and raw negative emotions to a different compartment. There are natural actors born to play the part—and there are those who need occasional prompting.

Physicians who are constitutionally unable to adopt the role on a regular basis and who persistently abrade the dignity of patients presenting for help—with all due respect to the specialty—ought to consider radiology.

Teaching Points

1. Dealing with depressed or psychotic patients often requires extreme patience. Expressing frustration is usually counterproductive.

2. Conduct telephone arguments out of the earshot of staff and patients.

3. Potentially derogatory comments about patients should be avoided in general. Even if spoken so that a patient cannot overhear, they create a negative atmosphere and legitimize similar behavior from other staff.

Case 7
Speaking of Empathy . . .

Quality Assurance Committee
Community Hospital
USA
Re: treatment of my daughter in your emergency room on January 24.

To Whom It May Concern:

This letter is being written in regards to the poor treatment my daughter and myself received while in your Emergency Room.

Let me first state that it was Friday, January 24 at 5:30pm when we entered the ER. We waited in the waiting room until approximately 7pm. We were then taken to a room and a nurse took down information. It was another 20 minutes before we were seen by the doctor. My daughter is 2½ years old. I will not even give him the satisfaction of addressing him as a physician, only perhaps a veterinarian, after the rough and inappropriate treatment she received. First off, he never introduced himself upon entering the room. Then I said, "Please excuse her for crying, she really hates hospitals," and his reply was, "Well we don't have time for this, get her to calm down, we're real busy."

I feel he was not only very rude but rough with my daughter. My daughter was in severe pain and his actions were very unjust and upset her even more. This man did not even spend two minutes looking at her. I truly find it appalling to have to pay $50 or more to wait over two hours to be seen by this individual, who spent two minutes in the room being totally unprofessional. Maybe I don't have a PhD behind my name, but I work full time, pay my bills, and expect proper treatment.

Due to the inappropriate treatment my daughter received, you've lost my business and my family's forever. It's too bad that one bad egg ruins it for your entire hospital. And believe me when I say this . . .
I will spread the word.

Sincerely,

Patient's Mother

CC: Hospital President, Chief of Staff, Chief of ER.

Several weeks later the emergency physician responded as follows:

Chairman of the Quality Assurance Committee
Community Hospital
USA

Dear Ms. Chairman,

I got the complaint letter you forwarded and here's my response. I remember the case well. The chart said the child might have a urinary tract infection. That's what the mother said, at any rate. The nurse's initial assessment was that there was a very red area on the vulva and groin. When I went into examine I took a nurse with me because I was concerned about possible child abuse. As I remember, we both introduced ourselves, and at any rate we were wearing name tags.

On entering the room the child immediately began screaming and crying. She was very difficult to examine. I questioned the mother about persons having contact with the child or possible burn accidents, and the way the child screamed also heightened my suspicion of possible abuse. It was only after close inspection of the area with the help of the mother, the nurse, and myself that it was possible to see that it was only a monilial infection and not a burn. I definitely spent longer than two minutes examining the child due to the difficulty.

I did not mention child abuse per se to the mother, but did ask questions germane to that possibility. Because we are state mandated to check for that, I could not avoid asking those questions. I wasn't aware the mother was upset. After the urinalysis came back negative, I went in, gave a prescription and they left. As far as the long wait goes, I had no control over that. It was a busy night.

Contact me if you need more information.

Yours sincerely,

Emergency physician

Analysis

Child abuse can present in subtle ways to the emergency department. Unless one keeps a high index of suspicion, it is all too easy to miss. Actually, the more common complaint coming across an emergency department director's desk is when a case of possible abuse was missed or not explored thoroughly enough.

One can only compliment the physician for being concerned about child abuse, but one element about his response to the complaint is striking. It seems quite clear from his description of events that he raised the issue of child abuse before trying to determine whether the patient's clinical findings might fit a pattern that should illicit this concern. He said that he did not tell the mother of his concern about child abuse but asked her questions to approach the subject. It is hard to see the difference. Granted, the triage nurse's assessment raised the issue of a possible burn. Was her assessment, however, sufficient evidence for acting when the patient was lying on the stretcher in front of him, awaiting his exam (albeit unhappily)?

All emergency physicians know from experience that it is emotionally difficult to broach the subject with patients or family members about the possibility of abuse, be it child, domestic, sexual, or elder abuse. Often health care providers are reluctant to offend in the event that a suspicion turns out to be unfounded. Nonetheless, we must do it—but only if there is sufficient reason for suspicion. The physician clearly should have looked before pursuing that line of questioning.

The fruit of such questioning—in the setting of a long wait and a physician who was busy and distracted and gave an impression of callousness—was an extremely upset mother and damage to the hospital's reputation.

Teaching Points

1. Physicians often walk a thin line between insult and appropriateness when dealing with parents who may be involved in abusive behavior with children.

2. It is always better to err on the side of asking embarrassing questions—but only if the situation warrants such concern.

Case 8
A Little Slip of the Tongue

A 35-year-old man complained that the emergency physician had violated the confidentiality of his medical records. The patient was a "frequent flyer" to the emergency department with headaches and back pains. He had long been perceived by nursing staff to be a drug-seeker, and they briefed the emergency physician on the patient's arrival. The emergency physician had never seen the man before. Before entering the room, he decided to read the patient's medical records, including his psychiatric file. The search was productive. He found a psychiatric evaluation from 6 years previously, indicating that the patient had undergone rehabilitation for substance abuse and had attempted suicide many years previously in a different state.

As the physician went to examine the patient, he first encountered the man's fiancée in the hallway. Seeing an opportunity to obtain additional history, he questioned the fiancée and in the process mentioned the patient's drug rehabilitation admission and suicide attempt.

Suffice to say, all of this was news to the fiancée, who promptly went into the room, confronted the patient, and broke off their relationship on the spot.

Over the next week, the patient placed numerous calls to the hospital to complain that his confidentiality had been violated. He also contacted an attorney more than willing to take the case.

Analysis

Although a pundit might say that the well-intentioned emergency physician inadvertently did the girlfriend a favor, there is no question that he breached the confidentiality of the patient's medical records. Negative outcomes included a substantial out-of-court settlement, a great deal of emotional distress to the patient, and collateral damage to the hospital's reputation.

All physicians find themselves at one time or another faced with making decisions about the degree to which they share information with friends, loved ones, or colleagues of a patient. Clearly we must take great care when dispensing negative information unearthed from a patient's past. Sometimes it may be appropriate and necessary to share such information, but only if the benefits to be gained clearly and obviously outweigh the risks. For example, if the patient had arrived comatose and the cause was still uncertain, to ask the fiancée about suicidal behavior and recent drug use in the context of the patient's past history would be clinically justifiable and worthy of legal defense.

The test, therefore, as to whether sensitive information should be shared without the patient's consent is whether it might yield information that would benefit the evaluation and treatment of the immediate clinical problem. In this particular case, the physician asked the patient's girlfriend whether he was still using cocaine. The question was appropriate: the patient had a headache, and cocaine use would put him at risk for intracranial hemorrhage. But there was no point in pursuing the issue when the girlfriend replied, "What do you mean, still using cocaine?"

This case illustrates a significant—and far more common—pitfall that awaits the emergency physician. The emergency department cannot function without emergency nurses. Most emergency physicians rely on them more than they realize. Many of us can give examples of being diverted from the wrong diagnostic or therapeutic pathway by the astute observations of an emergency nurse. But this sword cuts both ways. Most emergency physicians also can give examples of being misled by editorial comments such as, "This won't take you long, it's just an anxiety attack," or "Here she is again—same-old, same-old."

Such comments, often accompanied by cynical or condescending expressions, are common. Often they are accurate, but the wise physician considers these with a critical eye. Problems arise for emergency physicians when they allow themselves to be steered down this reductionist road. Physicians must bring to each patient's bedside a fresh, *inclusionist* attitude so that the full weight of their training and experience can be focused on the immediate situation, uncontaminated by externally generated prejudice. Easier said than done, but otherwise, things will be missed that should not be missed, or said that should not be said.

When the nurses briefed the physician about their belief that the patient was a manipulative drug-seeker, they were assigning him a certain position on the ladder of humanity and inviting the physician to do the same, sight unseen. This is the nurse's perogative. Our concern is the physician's response. If the same patient were a highly respected judge with the same distant history of substance abuse treatment and suicide attempt, most physicians would be highly sensitive, thoughtful, and circumspect about revealing negative history from a medical record.

The best approach lies in the old adage about treating every patient as if he or she were a family member—or a judge, for that matter. When an emergency nurse dismisses a patient, read between the lines.

Teaching Points

1. Carefully weigh the appropriateness of sharing confidential information with *anyone* without the patient's consent.

2. Try to eliminate subjective judgments about a patient based on appearance, nature of complaint, or "briefing" by a nurse.

3. Endeavor to treat every patient as you would want someone to treat your parent or your child.

Case 9
A Matter of No Little Weight

A 31-year-old woman who was 5 weeks pregnant presented to the emergency department one evening with the complaint of profuse vaginal bleeding that began in the afternoon. The next day she reported the following events in a conversation with the hospital quality assurance coordinator:

> The doctor went out of the room and half closed the door and began talking to a nurse about how he was not looking forward to doing a pelvic exam on me because of how large I am. He said it three or four times—that he'd never done a pelvic exam on someone this large and he wasn't even sure if he could do it. And he seemed to be making a joke about it.

The quality assurance coordinator said that the patient, who had been discharged with the diagnosis of spontaneous abortion, was crying during the conversation. She tried to calm the patient by telling her that the physician would want to apologize.

The patient then responded: "An apology would do no good even if he came to me personally because I would probably spit in his face. He should not be a doctor."

Analysis

Few physicians possess such purity of spirit as to have never uttered a derogatory comment toward a patient under their care. Many of us yield to the temptation from time to time, but usually in such a way as to spare the patient from our professional lapse. A miscarriage is a distressing, grief-provoking incident; in this case, it was made worse by an inexcusable lapse of discretion on the physician's part.

Teaching Points

1. Always be cognizant that comments made within earshot of patients and their family may be overheard. This is also true of patients who may appear unconscious.

2. A patient's sense of emotional well-being can be influenced positively or negatively by the caring and compassion a physician projects or fails to project.

3. Negative judgments of a patient's character or condition predispose to negative outcomes.

Case 10
I Told You So

A 27-year-old woman was watering rose bushes at a local nursery when a hornet stung the tip of her middle finger. After several minutes she began to feel lightheaded and nauseated. By the time she sat down in the break room, she noticed "blotches" on her arm and face. Her employer called 911, and EMTs transported the patient, herself a volunteer basic EMT, to the emergency department. On arrival at the emergency department, her vital signs were normal. The "blotches" had begun to fade, and after a leisurely triage she was left to wait in an examining room. Twenty minutes later, she stated, the emergency physician entered the room, looked at her chart and her finger, and said, according to the patient, "Why did you come here by ambulance for a little bee sting? You know that it costs over a hundred dollars? You just need some benadryl by mouth."

She replied that she had always come to the ED after bee stings in the past and that this was the worst reaction she had ever had. The physician had always given her a shot and pills stronger than benadryl.

She said that the emergency physician then seemed to become angry. He waved his finger at her, telling her he had been practicing for 10 years and ought to know how to treat her. She was not having a severe reaction and needed no other treatment—period.

At this point the patient stood up and strode out of the room, telling him as she passed that she was an EMT herself and did not appreciate his comments about misuse of the ambulance. Many times she had gotten up in the middle of the night to answer ambulance calls and never would she tell a patient what the physician told her.

The emergency physician, she said, followed her down the hall and asked to speak with her privately. He led her into the triage room, where he apologized and informed her that he was tired and going through a divorce and did not mean what he had said.

In the lengthy complaint letter she wrote to the hospital administrator, the patient said that she appreciated the physician's efforts to apologize and sympathized with his personal situation. In the meantime, she had gone to her family doctor and gotten a prescription for EpiPen. She said that even though the emergency physician had apologized, it did

23

not excuse his belittling her and suggested that he should either leave his personal issues at home or take a leave of absence.

The hospital administrator called the emergency department director and agreed with the patient's suggestion.

Analysis

Emergency physicians, like all clinicians, should try and educate their patients about the proper use of health care resources. But there is a time and a place for effective education, and there are better and worse ways to educate. Scolding may get the point across and relieve frustration on the part of the scolder, but it seldom has the desired effect, especially with adults, and it frequently generates a backlash of anger that is counterproductive.

Emergency physicians must deal with situations in which patients have either overreacted or underreacted to various situations, and questions about the quality of the patient's judgment or intelligence may arise in the physician's mind. Under the right circumstances, it is very easy for a little anger to blossom. That may be fine, as long as it does *not* translate into unprofessional comments.

As this case illustrates, once the physician stops exercising the nonjudgmental empathy that patients have every right to expect, the horse is out of the barn. After that point, asking the patient for forgiveness and sympathy usually serves only to widen the gap.

The key to avoiding this trap is to practice universal empathy. An old French proverb says it well: to understand all is to forgive all. Once the physician gets inside the patient's world, the patient's actions usually begin to make sense.

Empathizing with the patient also has another real benefit: *it is far easier and more effective to educate an ally.*

Teaching Points

1. It can be hard to practice empathy all of the time, but it is always worth the effort.

2. If there is a breakdown in communications between physician and patient, a simple apology is better than an attempt to rationalize a lapse of professionalism.

Case 11
Bothering Consultants

One of the hospital's billing clerks brought her husband into the emergency department on a busy Saturday afternoon. Mr. Jones had injured his right hand while operating a mechanical wood splitter. After a wait of about two hours, the emergency physician examined the patient's hand and noted that the distal pulp of the index finger had been partially avulsed, although it was still attached by a thick flap. The bone was not grossly exposed.

The physician ordered an x-ray and discovered that the distal tuft of the index finger had indeed suffered a fracture. She then asked the nurses to set up suturing equipment, went back into the room, and began to glove, whereupon, Mrs. Jones, the billing clerk, expressed surprise that the orthopedic surgeon was not being called. The physician informed her that this was a "routine injury" for which the orthopedic surgeon did not need to be bothered. Mrs. Jones pointed out that she had a personal relationship with the on-call orthopedist and felt that he should be involved. The emergency physician reiterated that it was not necessary and proceeded to repair the injuries. She debrided the injuries, sutured where necessary, administered antibiotics, and discharged Mr. Jones for follow-up with the orthopedist.

A week later, the repaired avulsion flap on Mr. Jones' index finger had become necrotic and subsequently sloughed. It was two months before he became fully functional at work again. Mrs. Jones demanded an interview with the hospital medical director to complain about the emergency physician's refusal to call Dr. A, the orthopedist. "It didn't look so busy to me. She had plenty of time to call. Every time I went out to the hallway, there she was sitting at the nursing station twiddling her thumbs."

Analysis

A thorough review of the case by the emergency department medical director indicated that the emergency physician had done a competent job and that consultation with the orthopedic surgeon was not mandatory. The debridement of fingertip amputations and avulsion lacerations, even in the presence of distal phalangeal fractures, is well within the scope of practice for emergency physicians. The complication of sloughing was not a sign of poor technique. There were, however, clear-cut signs that problems would arise. The emergency physician, who was a recent graduate of an excellent emergency medicine residency, admitted taking offense when Mrs. Jones called into question her competence to do the repair. She felt sure that it had more to do with the fact that she was female than anything else. She felt insulted and bullied and became determined to do what she knew was right.

The bottom line, of course, is that a successful outcome involves more than medical skill. Physicians must always address the expectations and concerns of patients and their families—no matter how unrealistic—or run the risk of losing the greater struggle. This physician should have swallowed her pride, sat down with Mrs. Jones, and explained the situation. If Mrs. Jones still persisted in requesting the surgeon, the physician at least should have placed a call. Such a call probably would have resulted only in his "blessing" to continue, but the compromise probably would have defused Mrs. Jones' frustration and paved the way to a positive encounter, wherein the complication would have been recognized for what it was—an unavoidable situation—rather than the result of incompetence.

By charging ahead, however, the emergency physician unfairly tarnished her reputation at the hospital.

Teaching Points

1. Physicians must always address the expectations and concerns of patients and their families—no matter how unrealistic.

2. This may mean calling for consultation when consultation is needed more for political than clinical reasons.

3. A satisfactory outcome always involves maintenance of a positive physician–patient relationship.

Case 12
The Ouch Factor

A 35-year-old man who was a frequent visitor to the emergency department for a variety of complaints had a history of anxiety disorder and was considered to be a potential drug-seeker. On the occasion in question, he presented a litany of new and old complaints, including headache, chest pain, chest itching, back pain, and intermittent swelling of his left wrist for several years. Within the past six months he had received negative rheumatologic and cardiac work-ups.

The emergency physician examined him, found nothing physically amiss, and felt compelled to order an EKG, which was normal. While waiting, the patient had made numerous requests to the nursing staff for a shot to help him feel better. The emergency physician discussed treatment options with a resident and decided to administer negative reinforcement. A nurse overheard the conversation, during which the emergency physician extolled the virtue of magnesium sulfate as being both nontoxic and extremely painful as an intramuscular injection. The emergency physician ordered the injection, and a little while later the patient was observed ambulating out the front door, muttering and rubbing his left buttock.

The next day an anonymous call was placed to the state health department about the ethics of using magnesium as negative reinforcement. Despite the retention of an excellent (and expensive) attorney to defend him, the emergency physician received a letter of censure from the state and was place under 12 months of monitored practice, during which the hospital invited him to seek employment elsewhere.

Analysis

The use of painful or noxious procedures or interventions of any kind as negative reinforcement has no place in clinical medicine. Because no studies demonstrate a benefit, the border between negative reinforcement and gratuitous cruelty is too fine to measure. Although this case was a gross example of inflicting unnecessary pain on a patient, other more subtle and common forms of negative reinforcement should be avoided as well. Examples range from the adoption of a severe and gruff manner toward an adolescent suicide gesture in hopes of "showing them it's not any fun" to the use of gastric lavage in a similar case when activated charcoal would have been perfectly adequate.

The endpoint of negative reinforcement is theoretical and nebulous at best and requires a moralistic judgment on the part of the physician that runs counter to the Hippocratic ethical stance of objective compassion toward all. Tough love may have its place among parents and judges, but not among physicians.

Teaching Points

1. Painful procedures for the sake of providing negative reinforcement or preventing patients from returning to the emergency department have no place in emergency medicine.

2. Avoid any kind of subliminal "patient teaching" that involves inflicting physical or psychological discomfort.

Case 13
A Systematic Review

By the reports of family, emergency medical technicians, and emergency department staff, Mr. Vincello was more than a little testy when he arrived one evening around midnight with multiple complaints, primarily shortness of breath and shakiness. He was a 63-year-old smoker with chronic obstructive pulmonary disease and hypertension. He did not hit it off with the emergency physician (EP), to say the least. The interchange between them, according to a couple of testimonials, follows:

EP: (strides into the room with his head down, reading the extensive chief complaint written by the nurse on the chart. Without introducing himself, he looks up and speaks, his voice cool and edged with frustration.)
So, why are you here tonight? Have you seen your doctor about these problems?

Patient: (seems taken aback, and hesitates for a moment. His eyes narrow.)
I would if it would do any goddamn good. My doctor's a quack. It's hardly worth going to see him.

EP: So you decided you'd be better of coming to the ED?

Patient: Why, are you a quack too?

EP: (tosses the chart on the counter, ungently.) All right, what's the main problem tonight? Just give me the main issue here.

Patient: I thought your job was to figure that out.

EP: Which is what I'm trying to do right now, sir.

Patient: Could have fooled me.

The interchange continued for several more minutes, according to spectators, and did not grow any more affectionate. The emergency physician did a brief exam and ordered a treatment of nebulized albuterol and atrovent, along with a chest x-ray and complete blood count. The patient's oxygen saturation, which initially had been 95% on room air, was 96% after the treatment. He was given a prescription for sulfamethoxazole-trimethoprim with underlined instructions to see his primary physician and discharged.

He returned to the emergency department, however, the following afternoon. His complaints were basically the same, although the weakness and shakiness were more prominent. The second emergency physician, after doing a more thorough review of systems than the first physician, ordered serum chemistries and discovered a blood glucose of 870 mg/dl. The patient was admitted with a diagnosis of new-onset type II diabetes mellitus.

While he was in the hospital, the patient and his family contacted the patient care representative and directed a complaint against the first physician on the basis of rudeness and incompetence.

Analysis

One of the frustrations of practicing emergency medicine involves dealing with patients who would have been better served by maintaining a good, active relationship with a primary care provider. This is especially true of elderly patients with multiple morbidities. There is no question that primary care providers can minimize the need for patients to visit emergency departments or become inpatients by screening for and aggressively managing chronic diseases. This ideal situation is far from universal. In the meantime, emergency physicians frequently deal with patients who carry a huge bag of complaints— some long-standing, some acute—with an expectation that the emergency physician will sort them out in a matter of 10 or 15 minutes. The fact is that many emergency physicians chose emergency medicine partly because of a lack of appetite for managing chronic problems. The mindset of most emergency physicians is geared toward resuscitation: a significant problem is simultaneously isolated, evaluated, and attacked. The patient with multiple complaints who does not appear grossly ill, however, requires a completely different and often much more time-consuming approach—a change of pace, if you will—that can be frustrating on a busy day because it often seems to lead nowhere.

But, frustration aside, such patients always present to emergency departments, and the emergency physician must adopt a strategy that will maximize efficiency and minimize the chance that something significant—such as incipient diabetes—will be missed. First of all, emergency physicians must banish as much as possible the impression of frustration or cynicism from their demeanor. Like this gentleman, some patients pick up on negative attitudes and may reciprocate. Once this occurs, the productivity and efficiency of subsequent communication may go out the window, and a frustrating situation may become an impossible one. The way to avoid this initial misstep is simply to give every patient all due respect and sympathy from the first moment of the encounter. Then, if the history of the present illness seems inordinately complex, focus instead on a good, thorough review of systems. This goal can be done quite adequately in less than five minutes. If the physician above had gone though a through review of systems, he quickly would have picked up on weight loss and appetite loss, not to mention polyuria and polydispsia. Even a first-year medical student at least would have checked the urine for glucose, and probably ordered a set of basic serum chemistries. Then, instead of being the subject of a major complaint and an embarrassing M&M rounds, the physician would have been a hero.

It also must be mentioned that on chart review, the nurse who triaged the patient tried to signal the physician that she felt that he was a bit of a crock. She had underlined the phrases: <u>too many complaints to register</u> and <u>admits to missing many appointments with his doctor.</u> This impression clearly helped to set the stage for what happened next—a breakdown in bedside manner.

Teaching Points

1. Complicated medical patients with multiple complaints who are noncompliant about visiting their primary doctors will always be a part of emergency medicine.

2. A good review of systems is worth its weight in gold for such patients.

3. The emergency physician must be wary of buying into the cynicism of providers who see the patient before they do.

4. Consider screening for diabetes and thyroid disorders in patients who present with confusing pictures.

Case 14
Comments Overheard

The following comments overheard by patients were extracted from complaint letters:

1. A 47-year-old patient with asthma was triaged into a treatment room on a busy day. After waiting an hour to see the physician, she rang the call bell. When the nurse responded, the patient reported increased trouble with breathing. The nurse went into the hallway, stopped the physician, and told him about the patient's situation. He said, "Don't worry; if she stops breathing, we'll just resuscitate her."

2. An elderly man with back pain had been waiting nearly two hours to see the physician. His granddaughter came out of the room and asked the physician (for the second time) when her grandfather would be seen. The physician replied that it would not be much longer and explained that they were having a terrible day. Then the physician added that the family always had the option to take the patient to a different hospital the next time.

3. A 35-year-old woman was en route to the emergency department by ambulance with chest pain. It was her second visit of the day. She had been diagnosed with chest wall pain and hyperventilation syndrome earlier that morning. The physician took the ambulance call and said, "Jesus Christ, not her again." This comment was overheard by the patient in the back of the rig.

Analysis

These three situations have five points in common:

1. They created distress for a patient.

2. They generated complaints that required a certain number of man-hours to resolve.

3. They made the entire ED staff look unprofessional.

4. They were utterly unnecessary.

5. Good clinical outcomes became bad public relations.

Emergency physicians often work in a frustrating environment, but venting in this fashion does not make the situation less frustrating. If the employees of Disney World and WalMart can learn the value of politeness, why cannot physicians?

Teaching Points

1. Avoid flippant or irreverent comments that may be overheard by patients.

2. It is probably best to avoid flippant or irreverent comments altogether. They set a tone for the entire department and, though initially a stress reliever, can eventually become toxic to morale.

Chapter 2

Case 15
Red Herrings

A 17-year-old girl, complaining of shortness of breath, was brought to the emergency department one afternoon by her mother. She had no cold or cough, and the onset of symptoms had been intermittent for about a week. She had recently started taking birth control pills. Her mother had taken her to see her family doctor three days previously. The family doctor diagnosed anxiety and referred the patient to a counselor, whom she had yet to visit.

The girl's respiratory rate was 28; her pulse, 116 beats/min; her blood pressure, 135/75 mmHg; and her oxygen saturation on room air, 96%. When the physician entered the room, she was breathing into a paper bag that the nurse had given her. He took her history and recorded that she was quite anxious. She did not have detectable wheezes on exam, but her expiratory phase seemed prolonged. The emergency physician ordered a treatment of nebulized saline and an oral dose of diazepam. After half an hour she reported feeling better and was discharged with instructions to follow-up with her primary care doctor if the symptoms did not resolve.

According to the patient's mother, the symptoms did not go away that evening. The next morning she took her daughter to a different emergency department, where blood gases were analyzed, followed by a lung scan. The diagnosis of pulmonary embolism was made. Several members of the patient's immediate family had problems with hypercoaguability. She was anticoagulated and did well.

But the patient's mother called hospital administration to complain that her daughter's evaluation in the ED was slipshod. She also changed family doctors.

Analysis

Because the range of symptoms associated with pulmonary embolism (PE) is wide and inconsistent, almost any person who presents to the emergency department with shortness of breath is a potential candidate for the diagnosis. This case illustrates how easy it is to become complacent. The usual 17-year-old who presents to the emergency department with shortness of breath and a clear chest is hyperventilating. As the physician admitted, the thought of a PE never entered his mind. This is understandable, since most emergency physicians will only see an adolescent PE case once or twice in their career. This case, thankfully, led to a complaint, not a suit for wrongful death.

But were there clues that might have led the physician to suspect more than just another adolescent anxiety attack? An oxygen saturation of 96% in a healthy 17-year-old with a clear chest should raise a clinician's eyebrows. It does not fit the picture of a hyperventilating teenager. Strange also was that fact that the patient's discharge vital signs still revealed tachypnea and a tachycardia of 110 despite the dose of diazepam. Based on these considerations, the patient deserved a set of blood gases. The next day at the second ED she had a pCO_2 of 32 mm Hg, a pO_2 of 86 mm Hg, and an A-a gradient of 23. These findings, in combination with the sinus tachycardia and tachypnea, triggered further evaluation.

The first emergency physician simply did not include PE in his differential diagnosis, an omission equivalent to putting on blinders.

Teaching Points

1. PE must be in the differential diagnosis of all patients who present with dyspnea.

2. Unexplained low oxygen saturation, tachypnea, and tachycardia—with or without chest pain or obvious risk factors—are sufficient to promote further consideration of the diagnosis.

3. Always exercise worst-case scenario thinking. Ask yourself the question—no matter how statistically unlikely, what is the worst problem that could affect the patient? Most of the time, simple clinical factors exclude "bad actors," but if we do not think of them up front, we may not think of them later.

Case 16
Fatal Miss

Mrs. Smith was an obese 49-year-old woman who presented to the emergency department one busy Sunday afternoon with a two-day history of feeling weak and experiencing some chest pain with breathing. She also complained of aching in her joints and a headache. She had no nausea, cough, sore throat, fever, or diarrhea. She had a history of hypertension and was taking hydrochlorothiazine and Premarin. She smoked a little over 1 pack per day. On admission to the emergency department, her oxyhemoglobin saturation was 97% on room air; her pulse rate, 100 beats/min; her respirations, 20 breaths/min; and her blood pressure, 170/92 mmHg. She was afebrile.

The emergency physician found no abnormalities on chest palpation or auscultation. She looked comfortable, but he decided, as he said later, to take a "fishing expedition" and ordered a complete blood count, chemistries, chest x-ray, and EKG. The EKG showed a slight sinus tachycardia and nonspecific ST changes. Her white blood cell count was normal, although she was a bit anemic. Her chest x-ray was normal. The only abnormal lab result was a potassium level of 3.1 mEq/L. The physician gave her a dose of oral potassium chloride and a prescription for more of the same. He then discharged the patient with diagnoses of hypokalemia and possible viral syndrome.

Mrs. Smith returned the following day in full arrest and expired in the emergency department. Autopsy revealed a massive PE.

Analysis

Such cases tend to be sobering for both experienced and novice emergency clinicians. They make us recall similar patients over whom we figuratively scratch our heads, while our pen moves to the chart and begins writing "possible viral syndrome."

What about this case should have signaled PE? We know that pleuritic chest pain is neither sensitive nor specific for PE. The emergency physician said that the patient described the pain so vaguely that he was not sure it even existed. Furthermore, the good oxygen saturation was reassuring. But how reassuring, actually, is pulse oximetry? Of all blood gas components, the partial pressure of oxygen is the least reliable indicator of a ventilation-perfusion mismatch because patients can increase pO_2 by increasing respiratory rate. The A-a gradient takes this into account, making it a more sensitive marker, although far from 100% sensitive or specific. Oxyhemoglobin saturation reflects only pO_2, which is marginally useful at best.

Given the patient's thromboembolic risk factors of obesity, smoking, and exogenous estrogen use, the normal oxygen saturation was not a reliable indicator. The patient deserved a blood gas evaluation. Although we can only speculate what the results would have shown, they might have led to further evaluation that may have saved her life. The sad fact is that the mortality rate for untreated PEs approaches 30%.

A more detailed discussion of evaluating for thromboembolic disease follows Case 18.

Teaching Points

1. Avoid overreliance on pulse oximetry results.

2. The decision to pursue a PE diagnosis must be based on an assessment of all aspects of the case—signs, symptoms, and risk factors.

3. Although not diagnostic for PE, arterial blood gas analysis can help to stratify risk and is much more useful than isolated pulse oximetry readings.

4. Always exercise worst-case scenario thinking. Keep the thought of PE in mind in any patient with pleuritic chest pain with or without dyspnea. All such patients will not require major investigations, but if the physician does not think of PE early, he or she may not think of it later.

Case 17
Breathing Freely

A 32-year-old woman came to the emergency department in the midmorning with shortness of breath, nausea, and diaphoresis. She felt as if she were going to pass out. She had no chest pain. Two weeks previously she had suffered a third-degree ankle sprain and was wearing a fiberglass short leg cast. Her pulse oximetry was 95% (she was a smoker); her pulse rate, 100 beats/min; her respiratory rate, 26 breaths/min; and her blood pressure, 118/79 mmHg. She had a history of asthma, panic attacks, and depression and was currently taking Prozac. She had used her albuterol metered-dose inhaler that morning without much relief of the dyspnea. Because of the leg immobilization, the emergency physician was concerned about the possibility of a pulmonary embolism. He ordered a battery of lab tests, including EKG, blood gases, complete blood count, serum chemistries, clotting studies, troponin level, and a ventilation-perfusion lung scan.

The EKG showed only a mild sinus tachycardia. The patient's pH was 7.41; her pCO_2, 34 mm Hg; and her pO_2, 90 mm Hg. The ventilation/perfusion (V/Q) lung scan was read as "low probability." All other lab tests came back normal. The emergency physician called the patient's primary doctor, discussed the case, and arranged for her to be seen in the office on the following morning. The emergency physician discharged the patient with a diagnosis of "hyperventilation syndrome."

The patient followed up with the primary care physician on the following day. No further tests were ordered. The primary physician reaffirmed the emergency physician's diagnosis of hyperventilation.

The next day, however, the patient returned to the emergency department in full cardiac arrest. Resuscitation efforts were unsuccessful. An autopsy revealed the cause of death to be a massive pulmonary embolism. There was also evidence of several smaller and slightly older pulmonary emboli.

The patient's family filed a complaint against both physicians with the state health department.

Analysis

Pulmonary embolism probably remains one of the most challenging diagnoses facing emergency physicians. In this a case the physician exercised worst-case scenario thinking and still missed the diagnosis. The problem, as borne out by many studies, is the lack of a single consistent clinical picture. Seldom does a patient present with the classic PE picture of acute pleuritic chest pain, shortness of breath, and hemoptysis.

The question in this case is as follows: given the patient's thromboembolic risk factor of leg immobilization, should the physician have felt comfortable stopping with just a low-probability V/Q scan? According to the PIOPED investigators, the answer would be no. In patients with a low-probability V/Q scan but high clinical suspicion for PE, the probability of disease remains about 14%.

The question then becomes, "Is the patient at high risk?" Unfortunately, as of yet there is no universal standard for classifying patients into definite low-, moderate-, and high-risk categories for PE. But, given the woman's leg immobilization, dyspnea, low pCO_2 (despite the normal pO_2 and normal A-a gradient* of 18), tachycardia, and tachypnea, most clinicians would put her into at least a high-to-moderate category, if not at high risk. The presence of leg immobilization as a risk factor carries great weight.

Given this analysis, a case can be made that the emergency physician should have gone beyond the normal lung scan for confirmatory testing.

Teaching Points

1. Clinical suspicion for PE must be based on a combination of symptoms, signs, risk factors, and lab values.

2. All tests for PE must be interpreted on the basis of pretest probability.

3. A normal VQ scan does not reliably exclude the diagnosis of PE in patients with moderate or high pretest probability for the disease.

4. Recent leg trauma and immobilization represent major risks for thromboembolic disease.

5. Untreated PEs carry a high risk of mortality.

---

*$P(A\text{-}a) = 150 - 1.25 \, pCO_2 + pO_2$. Upper limits of normal = 20.

Case 18
In the Crunch

A 47-year-old woman in otherwise excellent health developed chest pressure and severe shortness of breath while watching television about two weeks after undergoing open reduction and internal fixation of a trimalleolar fracture of her left ankle, which was still in a cast. Her husband called 911, and she arrived at the emergency department in marked respiratory distress. Despite oxygen administered by nonrebreather mask, she was cyanotic and diaphoretic, with a blood pressure of only 90/70 mmHg and a heart rate of 127 beats/min. She kept repeating to the medics, nurses, and the emergency physician who came into the room immediately after her arrival, "I need oxygen." No pulse oximetry was recorded in the chart, but a blood gas analysis demonstrated a pH of 7.45, a pCO_2 of 29 mm Hg, and a pO_2 of 57 mm Hg.

While awaiting the blood gas and portable chest x-ray results, the emergency physician evaluated another patient with suspected intra-abdominal injuries from a three-wheeler accident. Another seriously ill patient was receiving tissue plasminogen activator (tPA) for an acute myocardial infarction. It was ten minutes before he returned to the room—just in time to read the blood gas slip and notice that the patient had become unconscious and her breathing agonal. Her pulses were no longer palpable.

He immediately intubated the patient, and CPR was started. Resuscitation efforts continued without avail for another 45 minutes. Autopsy confirmed the presence of a massive PE. On the advice of a family friend (a physician), the patient's husband contacted the state health department and an attorney, concerned over why the patient had not been given a "clot buster" when she first arrived.

Analysis

Usually, when clinicians deal with PEs, the problem is diagnosis. In this case, the diagnosis was in little doubt. But would rapid administration of a fibrinolytic agent have truly helped, or was the patient doomed from the onset?

Before engaging in Monday morning quarterbacking, we must recognize that the emergency physician was dealing with other critical patients and felt unable to give the patient his undivided attention. That said, one point leaps out: the patient probably deserved immediate intubation. Despite maximal FiO_2 by mask, she bore clinical signs of severe hypoxia; in addition, she was hypotensive, suggesting that her cardiac reserve was already compromised. Immediate intubation and mechanical ventilation, combined with the use of vasopressors, would have bought some time. If a fibrinolytic agent had been administered, the fatal outcome may have been avoided, although we will never know for sure. Needless to say, by the time she arrested, it was too late for further intervention.

Based on the patient's presentation, the immediate use of a fibrinolytic agent would have been an appropriate consideration. The Food and Drug Administration has approved tPA (100 mg given over 2 hours) for this use, and a study has demonstrated its superior efficacy compared with heparin alone.[1] Another study involving small numbers of patients seems to demonstrate that streptokinase has equivalent efficacy.[2]

The patient appeared to have been a candidate for immediate airway control in anticipation of worsening respiratory and hemodynamic parameters. Without good initial airway control before a full arrest occurs, the clinician can fall too far behind to make a difference.

Teaching Points

1. Always consider immediate definitive airway control in patients who present in significant respiratory distress.

2. The use of fibrinolytic agents in patients with obvious pulmonary embolism accompanied by hemodynamic compromise may be life saving.

References

1. Goldhaber SZ, et al: Alteplase versus heparin in acute pulmonary embolism: Randomised trial assessing right-ventricular function and pulmonary perfusion. Lancet 341:507, 1993.
2. Meneveau N, et al: Comparative efficacy of a two-hour regimen of streptokinase versus alteplase in acute massive pulmonary embolism: Immediate clinical and hemodynamic outcome and one-year follow-up. J Am Coll Card 31:1057, 1998.

GENERAL DISCUSSION OF PULMONARY EMBOLISM DIAGNOSIS

As the previous four cases illustrated, few diagnoses in clinical medicine remain as problematic as pulmonary embolism (PE). This relatively common condition bears an inconsistent and often subtle clinical picture and, when untreated, may have a mortality rate as high as 30%. Therefore, it is not surprising that some of the most troubling cases to be presented at emergency medicine M&M rounds involve missed PE. It is clearly worthwhile to review in greater depth the state of the art for detecting PEs in emergency medicine.

1. **The value of various clinical factors and tests in evaluating for pulmonary embolism**

- Symptoms. The major symptoms of pulmonary embolism include pleuritic chest pain, dyspnea, anxiety, and syncope or near syncope. Unfortunately, these symptoms are highly nonspecific and relatively insensitive. They may be minimally present or absent altogether, although PE is uncommon in the absence of either dyspnea or chest pain.

- Clinical signs. The classic signs associated with acute PE include tachypnea (respiratory rate > 16 breaths/min); hemoptysis; tachycardia; hypotension; auscultatory changes of the chest, such as rales, wheezing, and rubs; and signs of right heart failure in cases of massive embolism. Signs associated with thromboembolic disease of the legs are present in less than half of patients. These factors are nonspecific and insensitive.

- Risk factors. Well-established risk factors for PE include immobilization, burns, hospitalization/bed rest, history of deep venous thrombosis or PE, stroke/spinal cord injury, hypercoagulable states (protein C deficiency, protein S deficiency, antithrombin III deficiency, malignancy), prolonged travel, pregnancy, recent surgery, trauma (especially lower extremity and pelvis), obesity, preexisting cardiac or pulmonary disease, and estrogen therapy.

- EKG and chest x-ray. The classic findings for PE of the qIII, tIII, S1 pattern on the electrocardiogram and a wedge-shaped infiltrate on the chest radiograph (the "Hampton hump") are insensitive diagnostic markers. The most common EKG findings in PE are sinus tachycardia and nonspecific ST changes. The primary value of both the EKG and chest x-ray is to exclude other conditions.

- Blood gas analysis. The classic PE pattern is a diminished pCO_2 (< 35 mm Hg), accompanied by a low pO_2 (< 80mm Hg), and an elevated A-a gradient (calculated at 150 minus 1.25 pCO_2 minus pO_2, with upper limits of normal at 20 mmHg). Numerous studies have confirmed that the sensitivity, specificity, and predictive value of any individual blood gas component in making the diagnosis of PE—with or without the addition of an A-a gradient calculation—are poor.[1,2] Blood gas values must be placed in the context of signs, symptoms, and risk factors.

- Ventilation/perfusion lung scanning. Numerous studies indicate that a significant percentage of patients with low-probability radioisotope lung scans have PEs. The miss rate rises as high as 20% or more in patients with high clinical suspicion of PE.[3-6] For this reason, a low-probability V/Q scan must be combined with clinical factors and cannot be used alone to exclude the presence of PE. Even lung scans read as completely normal can miss PE involving subsegmental branches of the pulmonary arterial circulation.

- Ultrasonography of the lower extremities. In perhaps 50% of patients with PE, lower leg thromboembolic disease is demonstrable on ultrasonography examination. Thus, a number of authors have proposed paradigms in which ultrasonography of the legs is used in combination with other tests to help make therapeutic decisions in potential PE patients.[7-9]

- Contrast-enhanced helical CT scanning. In recent years over two dozen studies have attempted to define the value of contrast-enhanced CT in the evaluation of PE. One point is clear: CT is not a diagnostic panacea that can reliably exclude the need for anticoagulation. Although it appears to have a high specificity (i.e., when positive, it pinpoints the diagnosis well), CT suffers from the same sensitivity limitation that plagues ventilation perfusion scanning.[10] Its rate of false negatives, especially for finding small PEs involving subsegmental branches, appears to be significant. A patient with an intermediate or high clinical probability of PE and a negative CT requires further testing, such as angiography.

- D-dimer. D-dimer is a fibrin degradation product. It is highly specific for PE, but because it is elevated in other conditions, especially cancer, its specificity for thromboembolic disease is poor. Two categories of D-dimer assays are available for clinical use at this time. One is a rapid latex agglutination test; the other is a more time-consuming enzyme-linked immunosorbent assay (ELISA). Most authors state that the latex agglutination test does not appear to be sufficiently accurate to warrant a role in the emergency department.[11] The ELISA assay, however, is used at many centers. Given its reasonable sensitivity and negative predictive value, many authors agree that a negative ELISA D-dimer assay in a low probability patient can be used to exclude the diagnosis of PE or DVT.[12] However, one also must accept the fact that, because of its low specificity, there are a fair number of false positives, which mandate further testing. ELISA D-dimer, therefore, is only a screening test, not a diagnostic modality.

- Pulmonary angiography. Angiography is the gold standard for diagnosing PE. Although it is an invasive procedure, it has a lower rate of complications than empirical anticoagulation.

2. A simple approach to the patient with a possible PE

The first step in diagnosing PE obviously lies simply in suspecting the diagnosis. But, given the wide range of symptoms, the highly variable clinical picture, and the broad age spectrum involved, it is sometimes easy not to think of PE. The 17-year-old girl in Case 15 exemplifies this problem. Although most 17-year-olds who present to the emergency department with shortness of breath have hyperventilation or asthma, this patient had an unexpectedly low oxygen saturation without the presence of wheezing, accompanied by a persistent relative tachycardia, and was taking birth control pills. PE was certainly in the differential diagnosis. Based on her age and lack of other risk factors, she was a low-probability patient, but she deserved at least an analysis of blood gases. If the gases were perfectly normal, she would have been an extremely low probability case, and, in all likelihood, most physicians would stop at this point. But, if blood gas and A-a gradient abnormalities had strengthened the suspicion, further evaluation would have been in order. In other words, she would have become a low-to-intermediate probability patient. As the physician admitted, the thought of PE never entered his mind. She was "too young." A subjective impression or prejudice interfered with his assessment of the empirical evidence. The point is simply to approach patients with as broad a differential diagnosis as possible.

An excellent article by Gallagher discusses a flexible algorithm for diagnosing PE that may involve any one test or any rational combination of the various tests at the physicians disposal: ELISA D-dimer, ultrasonography, V/Q scanning, helical CT, and angiography.[13] The physician must begin by categorizing the patient as low, moderate, or high probability based on assessment of clinical factors, although there is no universally accepted definition of these terms at present. An example of a low-risk patient, however, is a young person with pleuritic chest pain but normal chest x-ray and EGK and blood gases that show only a slight decrease in pO_2, with no significant risk factors. Conversely, a high-risk patient may have pleuritic chest pain, low pCO_2 and pO_2, elevated A-a gradient, history of prolonged bed rest after a lower extremity fracture, and normal chest x-ray.

Categorization is essential because the meaning of test results varies as a function of pretest probability. In low-probability patients, the physician may start by ordering an ELISA D-dimer (at this time, D-dimer should be limited to low-probability patients) or a lung scan. If the D-dimer is negative or the lung scan normal, PE can safely be ruled out. If the D-dimer is positive, however, or the lung scan "indeterminate," further work-up is necessary. Only a high-probability lung scan is sufficient grounds to begin anticoagulation therapy.

If further work-up is needed, the physician may choose to order ultrasonography of the legs. However, because 20% or more of PE cases have normal venous ultrasounds, the test is useful only if positive. A negative ultrasound warrants further evaluation.

The physician may choose to order a contrast-enhanced spiral CT of the chest. Like ultrasound of the legs, the spiral CT scan is most useful when positive. It appears to have a substantial rate of missing smaller, peripheral PEs. The miss rate may be acceptable in low-probability patients, but in patients with moderate or high probability of PE, a negative chest CT is not reliable to exclude the diagnosis. Angiography should be considered.

The general theme of this approach is that, with the exception of angiography, a negative test in the presence of moderate or high clinical probability tends to force the clinician toward further testing, and this principle becomes sounder in proportion to an increase in clinical suspicion. Which test to begin with depends, therefore, on clinical judgment in concert with available resources. The clinician must always keep in mind that empirical anticoagulation appears to carry a greater risk of complication than pulmonary angiography.

References

1. Stein PD, et al: Arterial blood gas analysis in the assessment of suspected acute pulmonary embolism. Chest 109:78, 1996.
2. Jones JS, et al: Use of the alveolar-arterial oxygen gradient in the assessment of acute pulmonary embolism. Am J Emerg Med 16:333, 1998.
3. PIOPED investigators: Value of the ventilation/perfusion scan in acute pulmonary embolism. JAMA 263:2753, 1990.
4. Worsley DF, et al: A detailed evaluation of patients with acute pulmonary embolism and low- or very-low-probability lung scan interpretations. Arch Intern Med 154:2737, 1994.
5. Stein PD, et al: Diagnostic utility of ventilation/perfusion lung scans in acute pulmonary embolism is not diminished by pre-existing cardiac or pulmonary disease. Chest 100:604, 1991.
6. Hull RD: The low-probability lung scan: A need for change in nomenclature. Arch Intern Med 155:1845, 1995.
7. Goodman LR, et al: Diagnosis of acute pulmonary embolism: Time for a new approach. Radiology 199:25, 1996.
8. Meyerovitz MF, et al: Frequency of pulmonary embolism in patients with low-probability lung scan and negative lower extremity venous ultrasound. Chest 115:980, 1999.
9. Stein PD, et al: Strategy that includes serial noninvasive leg tests for diagnosis of thromboembolic disease in patients with suspected acute pulmonary embolism based on data from PIOPED. Arch Intern Med 155:2101, 1995.
10. Rathburn SW, et al: Sensitivity and specificity of helical computed tomography in the diagnosis of pulmonary embolism: A systematic review. Ann Intern Med 132:227, 2000.
11. Farrell S, et al: A negative simplified D-dimer assay result does not exclude the diagnosis of deep vein thrombosis or pulmonary embolus in emergency department patients. Ann Emerg Med 35:121, 2000.
12. Perrier A, et al: Non-invasive diagnosis of venous thromboembolism in outpatients. Lancet 353:190, 1999.
13. Gallagher EJ: Clots in the lung. Ann Emerg Med 35:181, 2000.

Chapter 3

Doctor to Doctor
Communication Failures in the
Emergency Department

Case 19
The Reluctant Attending

A 46-year-old man came to the emergency department one morning after a night of nausea and vomiting, accompanied by numerous episodes of black diarrheal stools. Other than a history of a GI bleed some 10 years ago, he was healthy and taking no medications. The patient said that his vomitus had contained no obvious blood.

On examination he was afebrile, his pulse rate was 68 beats/min, and his blood pressure was 120/63 mmHg. The emergency physician wrote that he appeared to be in no acute distress. He was not pale. The nausea had subsided. His abdomen was soft and nontender, with good bowel sounds. Dark-colored fecal material in the rectal antrum on digital exam tested positive for occult blood. The emergency physician ordered a liter of normal saline IV and routine lab tests.

The white blood cell count was 6900/μl with a left shift of the differential, and the hemoglobin and hematocrit levels were 12.3 gm/dl and 41%, respectively. Blood urea nitrogen was 38 mg/dl; creatinine was 0.9 mg/dl, and serum electrolytes were normal, as were urinalysis and an abdominal free-air series. The patient, meanwhile, was tolerating sips of liquids but had had an additional stool that appeared melanotic and was strongly heme-positive. The emergency physician ordered an intravenous dose of an H_2 blocker and called the patient's primary physician to recommend admission.

The primary physician, however, happened to be one of the hospital's "iron gates." He chided the emergency physician for wanting to admit a stable patient who could just as easily be evaluated on an outpatient basis. He told the emergency physician to give him another liter of fluid, continue the H_2 blocker, and have him come to the office on the next day.

The emergency physician reluctantly agreed and approximately 1 hour later discharged the patient. At home, however, the melanotic diarrheal stools continued, and the patient had a syncopal episode.

He returned to the emergency department, where he was admitted. Endoscopy revealed an actively bleeding duodenal ulcer.

The patient's sister-in-law was one of the hospital's nurse managers. She filed a complaint with the medical director about the failure to admit the patient initially. According to her, at the time of discharge the patient was sweaty and, when he tried to stand up, became woozy. Nonetheless, he was hustled out the door.

When the chart was reviewed, no discharge vital signs could be found, and orthostatic blood pressures had not been measured. The primary physician stated that if he had known how sick the patient looked, he would not have recommended discharge: "But listen, that was the emergency doc's call, not mine."

Analysis

Emergency physicians like to believe that they practice in a collegial environment and that when they make decisions in concert with other physicians, they will receive all due professional respect and support. But not everyone plays by these rules. It is extremely easy, when a decision to discharge backfires, for the admitting physician simply to point out the truth: he was not the one looking at and touching the patient.

The emergency physician later admitted that he was not at all comfortable with discharging this patient—he had a gut sense that the man would be back. But the situation was somewhat equivocal, and it is true that not all GI bleeders need admission. He did not want the internist to think that he was a "wimp," misusing resources and afraid to send anybody home.

He also admitted that he did not personally evaluate the patient before his discharge, nor did he order orthostatic blood pressure measurements. Had he known that the man had become lightheaded and sweaty on standing up, he would have called the internist and demanded either admission or personal discharge of the patient by the internist.

Fortunately, the patient did well. However, if he had been at risk for cardiovascular complications, the hypotensive syncopal event at home could have had more serious sequelae beyond simply tarnishing the emergency physician's reputation.

Teaching Points

1. Reluctant admitting physicians add to the pressures of working in the emergency department, but their reticence should not color the emergency physician's judgment.

2. When a disagreement about patient disposition arises, the emergency physician retains the right to request (i.e., demand) that the admitting physician come and personally evaluate a patient that the emergency physician feels should be admitted.

3. Always carefully reevaluate all patients whose condition may become less stable after they leave the emergency department.

Case 20
Unsafe to Send

A 43-year-old woman with cerebral palsy, profound mental retardation, and an extensive history of coronary artery disease was transported to the emergency department with fever, cough, and shortness of breath. Her temperature was 103° F rectally; her pulse rate, 114 beats/min; her blood pressure, 105/58 mmHg; and her oxygen saturation, only 90% on 2 liters of oxygen by nasal cannula. The patient did not have do-not-resuscitate orders on file.

The emergency physician evaluated her immediately on arrival. He suspected pneumonia and ordered a chest x-ray and routine lab tests, including blood cultures. When the x-ray confirmed a pulmonary infiltrate, the physician ordered intravenous antibiotics. He had already placed the patient on 50% oxygen by a venturi mask, which led to stabilization oxygen saturations in the mid nineties. Meanwhile, the patient's systolic blood pressure began drifting below 100 mm Hg. But it responded well to saline fluid boluses.

It was an extremely busy day. Knowing that the patient was septic, the emergency physician quickly called the admitting physician, who happened to be in house, and who promptly evaluated the patient and arranged an ICU admission.

The lab results showed a white blood cell count of 19,500/µl with a marked left shift of the differential. BUN and creatinine levels were 40 mg/dl and 2.1 mg/dl, respectively, and serum potassium was critically high at 7.2 mEq/L. The emergency physician ordered a repeat potassium assessment for confirmation, then personally informed the admitting physician of the potassium levels.

The emergency physician returned to dealing with a number of other ill patients in the department; the admitting doctor spent approximately half an hour at the patient's bedside and reviewed labs and old records. The repeat potassium test came back at 7.2 mEq/L, confirming the existence of significant hyperkalemia.

At some point, the admitting doctor received a call from the bed supervisor to say that the last ICU bed had just been taken. The pneumonia case in the emergency department would need to be transferred. The admitting doctor sought out the emergency physician and told him of this unfortunate logistic complication during a 5-second conversation in the hallway.

Now the crux arises. The emergency physician assumed, based on previous experiences with the admitting physician, that the admitting physician would help arrange the woman's disposition and transfer; this time, however, the assumption was false. The admitting doctor had figuratively washed his hands of the case, leaving no documentation.

Half an hour later the charge nurse asked the emergency physician about disposition of the patient. The emergency physician located an accepting physician at a different hospital, filled out the COBRA paperwork, called an advanced life support unit to make the transport, reviewed the patients' vital signs one final time, and returned to seeing new patients.

Halfway to the receiving hospital, however, the patient went into ventricular fibrillation. She did not respond to defibrillation or medication in the ambulance and arrived at the second emergency department with CPR in progress. She was subsequently pronounced dead.

The ED staff at the receiving hospital reviewed her chart and discovered the two elevated potassium levels along with the fact that no treatment had been initiated. Furthermore, prearrest rhythm strips displayed marked QRS complex widening and premature ventricular contractions, suggesting that the elevated potassium level directly contributed to cardiac arrest.

A COBRA/EMTLA violation on the basis of insufficient stabilization before transport was declared and pursued to its usual ugly conclusion.

Analysis

The physician was a resident trained in emergency medicine at a fine program, widely acknowledged to be one of the best clinicians in the group. He had made a reasonable assumption that the admitting doctor would help out, given the obvious chaos in the emergency department. The patient was, after all, his. He made a second assumption that the admitting physician, cognizant of the hyperkalemia, would address it. But he failed to confirm that assumption, and the admitting doctor was under no obligation to help. No formal transfer of responsibility had taken place, and matters can slip from our minds.

The presence of the admitting doctor in the emergency department served to distance the emergency physician from the patient and to lessen his sense of responsibility and vigilance but did not relieve him of any responsibility. The admitting doctor should have helped, but that argument carried only a moral and no technical weight.

At the end of the day, the emergency physician's name was on the transfer papers—the buck stopped with him.

Teaching Points

1. COBRA/EMTALA regulations state that the patient must be adequately stabilized before transfer so that the risks of transfer do not outweigh the benefits.

2. The presence of an admitting physician in the emergency department caring for a patient can blur the lines of responsibility in ways potentially dangerous for the patient.

3. Be cautious of making assumptions about the transfer of responsibility while the patient remains in the ED. Unless it is in writing, the patient probably is still yours.

Case 21
Atypical Chest Pain

A 49-year-old woman presented to the emergency department with the chief complaint of several weeks productive cough and some chills. She also complained—at least to the nurse—of a burning sensation in her right chest. Her history included the fact that she had undergone angioplasty during the previous year and still smoked 1 pack of cigarettes per day. Her vital signs on admission to the ED were normal. She was afebrile, and her oxygen saturation was 96% on room air.

Based on the productive cough and pulmonary ronchi, the emergency physician diagnosed acute bronchitis. His notes on the chart stated that the patient denied chest pain or nausea and on exam showed no signs of congestive heart failure. He did not, however, mention the "burning" sensation described by the nurse. He elected not to order lab tests, chest x-ray, or EKG but prescribed a course of antibiotics and discharged the patient.

Three days later she returned by ambulance with crushing substernal chest pain accompanied by sweating and nausea. The EKG done on arrival was now consistent with an acute anterior wall infarction. She was quickly started on fibrinolytic therapy. Her pain did not resolve, and she was transferred several hours later to a tertiary care center, where angioplasty and stent placement were performed. When she left the tertiary care center 8 days later, she had poor residual left ventricular function.

The patient called the emergency department to complain. She said that her quality of life had diminished because of the heart attack and that the first physician had "dropped the ball." She was considering talking to an attorney.

Analysis

On initial review of the chart, it appears that the first physician's handling of the case fell within the standard of care. He documented a head-to-toe exam and complete history. He specifically noted that the patient denied chest pain, nausea, and diaphoresis, although he did not mention the patient's complaint of a burning feeling in her chest, which the nurse's note documented. In a brief sentence at the bottom of his note, he wrote that the patient's signs and symptoms pointed toward an upper respiratory infection. A second reviewer also felt that the physician's behavior did not deviate from the standard of care.

But might there have been a different outcome if the physician had done an EKG on the first visit? It is impossible to know for sure, but one point became clear in the patient's conversation with the emergency department director. She stated that when the doctor asked her about chest pain, she did not think of the burning sensation as a "pain" per se. She did recall, however, asking him if her symptoms may be coming from her heart. "Why didn't he think of that?" she asked.

Several issues bear discussion. First, the emergency physician's index of suspicion must always be high in patients with major cardiac risk factors. Cardiac chest pain can be all over the board in terms of quality and location. Classically it is like an intense pressure, but it can range from a light pressure to a dull ache or sharper sensation, or it can be nonexistent. "Did you have any chest *discomfort?*" is a much better way to phrase the question. It casts a finer net into the murky water of subjective sensations when you are trying to catch a slippery symptom. If the physician had used that type of query, he may have gone into more detail about the "burning" sensation—perhaps to the point of raising true concern. Studies show that cardiac pain in women is more likely to be atypical. One point is certain: when a complaint is missed or misunderstood, the onus lies with the physician, not the patient. Emergency physicians especially, given the mere seconds that we sometimes have to establish rapport and understand a patient's communication patterns, must become expert at ferreting out potentially significant symptoms.

Secondly, emergency physicians are sometimes accused of wasting lab tests and CTs on relatively trivial complaints. There is a growing pressure on all physicians to be more cost-effective. Clearly, many of the tests that we order almost by rote sometimes are unnecessary, such as urine cultures in healthy females with lower urinary tract infections. This particular physician had a reputation for not wasting tests, and he stated that in this case avoiding waste was his aim. On the other hand, the patient had a major set of risk factors and some chest discomfort and expressed her concerns to the doctor. At a minimum an EKG would have had great reassurance value, especially given the burning sensation and the potential to yield important diagnostic information. If the EKG had been positive, she might have received an earlier intervention. A negative EKG probably would have prevented the patient from living with the gnawing idea that a physician's mistake had shortened her life.

Although one can argue that the physician practiced within the standard of care and made no horrific mistake, I argue that the standard of care is merely a baseline. Above this baseline lies the "art of medicine."

Finally, the issue of dealing with patients who call or write to complain deserves a brief discussion. Perhaps in response to a system of training that involves years of having their behavior continuously and rigorously scrutinized and corrected by those higher in the pecking order, many physicians react with anger and defensiveness when faced with criticism from laypeople, especially when it seems petty and unfounded. This is sometimes true also of emergency department medical directors, who must respond to complaints against member of their staff. A tendency to circle the wagons can arise. Patients quickly sense this response, however, and the situation deteriorates. In general, any effort to explain to a patient or family member why their complaint is unfounded feels like an act of condescension. Their anger cannot be denied; it can only be listened to, accepted, and understood. Patients understand that physicians are subject to human failings, but when their complaints are handled with any trace of condescension or arrogance, this understanding does not come into play. On the other hand, when they are given a sympathetic forum in which to ventilate their feelings, they can begin moving beyond the immediate anger and may even spontaneously express a certain degree of forgiveness. Denying patients the right to be angry only fans the fire.

In general, detailed explanations of why a physician did or did not do something are not helpful unless the patient is suffering from complete misapprehension of the event. Even then, the person dealing with the complaintant must choose the right time to launch into an explanation. Establish a sympathetic rapport first. The danger lies in giving the impression of brushing off the patient's concern.

It is generally best not to have the physician involved in the initial contact with a complaining patient. The meeting can be extremely awkward for both parties and may be counterproductive. In many cases, the medical director is the first person to contact the patient and can play the role of mediator. In some cases, a response from the physician—in the form of a letter or a call—may be appropriate, but only after the situation has been assessed and all parties have had time to cool off. The most appropriate response to all complaints, however, is a mixture of sincere concern, sympathy, and perhaps explanation. The patient must be thanked for having brought the concern forward and be reassured that the matter will be dealt with quickly and appropriately. An apology for the patient's distress is always in order, but admissions of guilt and responsibility should be avoided. Attempts should be made to follow-up the complaint with a letter, call, or, in some cases, a personal meeting once investigations have been completed.

Responding with sensitivity and sincere concern to a patient's complaint can nip potential litigation in the bud. By calling the hospital before contacting an attorney, a patient has clearly signaled his or her desire to achieve emotional instead of legal redress. Physicians ignore, dismiss, or deny the validity of complaints at their own peril.

A patient must be told that his or her complaints will be used to improve the emergency department's service. As regrettable as complaints may be, they are golden opportunities for medical directors to reach into the community and to educate specific physicians and the group in general.

Rare is the complaint that cannot be turned into a lesson.

Teaching Points

1. Remember to document carefully a complete history and physical exam in every patient chart.

2. Always consider myocardial infarction when risk factors exist in a sick patient, especially:

- Women (presentation of myocardial infarction often atypical)

- Diabetics (neuropathy causes silent ischemia)

- Elderly patients (poor pain localization and barriers to expressing themselves)

3. Consider the cost/benefit ratio of a relatively inexpensive test, such as an EKG.

4. Make every attempt to address a complaint personally and respectfully, both to improve patient satisfaction and to reduce litigation claims.

Case 22
Why a Gastrointestinal Cocktail?

A 42-year-old man with chest pain presented to the emergency department by ambulance. The pain was partially epigastric and partially substernal and radiated somewhat to the left scapular area. He had been given three nitroglycerin tablets sublingually by the medics in the field without significant relief of discomfort, which had started just after lunch. He was not nauseated, short of breath, or sweaty but was belching frequently. His history was significant for a minor cerebrovascular accident the year before and angioplasty 2 years previously. He also had a history of gastroesophageal reflux disease (GERD) and hypertension and was currently taking Procardia, omeprazole, and an occasional nitroglycerin tablet. His family history was highly positive for cardiac disease, and the patient still smoked a pack and a half of cigarettes per day.

When the emergency physician examined the patient, his pain was still rated at 3 out of 10, but he looked comfortable and in no acute distress. His vital signs were unremarkable. His chest was clear, and his cardiovascular exam was normal, but he had mild tenderness in the epigastric region. The nurse handed the physician an EKG, which showed a normal sinus rhythm at 96 beats/min and some minor-appearing, nonspecific abnormalities.

Given the patient's epigastric tenderness, the belching and the history of GERD, the physician elected to give him a gastrointestinal (GI) cocktail before trying more nitrates. Meanwhile, lab samples were drawn, and a portable chest x-ray was taken. Five minutes later, the emergency physician returned to the room and discovered that the patient was pain-free. The GI cocktail seemed to have worked. The chest x-ray was normal, and all lab tests, including troponin level, were normal. The emergency physician obtained an old chart and discovered that the nonspecific EKG changes were chronic. He checked on the patient and did a rectal exam, which was negative for occult blood. He contacted the patient's primary physician, discussed the case, and told the physician that in his opinion the patient's symptoms were probably GI. The primary physician agreed, and the patient was discharged, still pain-free, after a total stay of approximately three hours.

On the drive home, however, the patient developed chest pain that rapidly became severe, accompanied by nausea and diaphoresis. His family, disappointed that he had not been admitted in the first place, drove directly to a different emergency department 20 miles away, where he was admitted with unstable angina and underwent triple bypass surgery several days later.

The patient's wife called the hospital administrator to inform him of the emergency physician's mistake. Earlier she had contacted the primary physician and was told that he had not recommended admission because the emergency room doctor did not share the entire story.

Analysis

So much for collegiality. Although involving a patient's primary doctor in difficult disposition decisions is always an excellent idea, it will not shield the emergency physician from criticism when the final decision is questionable. Was the emergency physician's decision to send the patient home justifiable? It has long been a truism that subjective relief after a GI cocktail is neither sensitive nor specific for excluding cardiac causes for pain. The results of a GI cocktail must be weighed against other factors—in this case, the presence of an extremely high-risk profile. In the end, each case must be decided on the basis of many variables, but most experienced physicians (i.e., those who have been led astray in the past) do not give much credence to what the GI cocktail seems to be saying. At the end of the day, it is really a matter of probability and risk factors.

Teaching Points

1. Do not take much assurance from pain relief by a GI cocktail in patients with significant cardiac risk factors. The results are too unreliable, and too much is at stake.

2. Err on the side of safety for the patient, and consider banishing the GI cocktail from your diagnostic armamentarium.

3. Admitting physicians like to be called about patients whom you do not believe need to be admitted. They will seldom try and talk you out of sending a patient home. The end game is yours.

Case 23
A Tooth for a Truth

A 72-year-old woman presented to the emergency department with a toothache. It woke her up the night before, had been intermittent for two days, and was becoming worse. She made an appointment with her dentist for next week. She had a history of hypertension and diet-controlled diabetes. She was triaged to the fast track and seen in a timely fashion by the physician on duty. Her vital signs were normal. Examination revealed no tender teeth on percussion, although she did seem somewhat tender at the left temporomandibular joint (TMJ). The pain also seemed vaguely related to opening and closing of the jaw, although the physician later admitted that the patient was highly equivocal on this point.

The emergency physician prescribed ibuprofen and discharged the patient with a tentative diagnosis of TMJ syndrome vs. early dental infection.

Three hours later the patient collapsed at home and was brought into the emergency department in full arrest. She could not be resuscitated. Autopsy revealed significant coronary artery disease with severe narrowing of the left anterior descending artery and changes consistent with recent myocardial infarction. An attorney for the patient's family contacted the hospital several weeks later, and a settlement was ultimately made on behalf of the patient.

Analysis

It was clear from talking with the physician, who was a well-trained family doctor working in the emergency department's fast track, that a cardiac cause for the patient's symptom had never crossed his mind. The case seemed straightforward. He did not perform a full review of symptoms and did not ask about the relationship of the pain to exertion, nor about the presence of associated symptoms. The patient—whose complaint also failed to set off any alarms in the mind of a battle-tested triage nurse—did not volunteer such information.

This case serves as a reminder to all physicians that cardiac ischemia can present as isolated pain in the jaw. Physicians must maintain a high index of suspicion, especially in patients more likely to have atypical cardiac presentations—diabetics and women.

Teaching Points

1. Always practice worst-case scenario thinking. If a condition is not considered up front, it may never be considered in the differential diagnosis.

2. *Every* patient who presents with a toothache should elicit in the physician's mind at least a passing concern that the pain may be of cardiac origin. Usually, of course, their worry can be laid to rest almost immediately by exam and history.

3. Remember the truism that atypical presentations of cardiac disease are more common in women and diabetics.

4. Never assume that patients triaged to a fast track may not have major problems. Until triage is perfect, such errors will occur.

Case 24
Taking the EKG to Heart

A 71-year-old woman presented to the emergency department with complaints of mild flu-like symptoms with a cough for several days. The cough was productive of yellow sputum, and she also reported intermittent pain in her upper chest. In addition, she had a sore throat and loss of appetite. There was no vomiting or diarrhea with her flu-like symptoms, although she did complain of some nausea. Her past history was significant for hypertension, hiatal hernia, angina, and non–insulin-dependent diabetes. Her current medications, other than a daily aspirin, were unknown; the nursing note referred to a list, which at some point must have become separated from the chart.

The emergency physician evaluated the patient. Her vital signs were normal, expect for a mildly elevated blood pressure and a heart rate of 101 beats/min. Her chest exam was remarkable for the presence of mild bilateral ronchi, perhaps more prominent at the left base. Her heart tones were normal with no signs of cardiac failure. Her membranes were pink and moist, and her abdomen soft and nontender. The emergency physician ordered routine lab tests and a chest x-ray.

The chest pain was a major concern. It had begun several hours before admission, radiated to the left shoulder, and lasted perhaps an hour. The patient, however was not a good historian. But given her history of diabetes and angina, the physician decided to order an EKG and troponin level.

The patient's blood work, including troponin level, was normal, as was her chest x-ray. The emergency physician interpreted the EKG as showing a normal sinus rhythm at 90 beats/min with no significant changes. There were no further episodes of chest pain. He discharged the patient with a prescription for a 5-day course of antibiotics and a diagnosis of bronchitis and flu-like syndrome.

On the next day the emergency department received a call from the patient's primary care doctor. The patient had just been admitted from his office. She had presented with chest pain and now had EKG changes consistent with an inferior myocardial infarction. He had just received a copy of the patient's chart, along with a copy of her EKG. He inquired what was going on: If the emergency physician was suspicious of a cardiac cause, why had he discharged her after performing only a single troponin level?

That was a question that the quality improvement committee asked as well.

Analysis

Troponin levels generally do not begin rising until 4–6 hours after an ischemic event and may not rise significantly, if at all, in preischemic coronary syndromes. If a patient comes to the emergency department 6 or more hours after an episode of chest pain, it may be reasonable to obtain a single troponin level. A negative level may be factored into the clinical decision making. However, if the pain began less than 6 hours before admission—or if unstable angina is a concern—a single troponin level is worthless. It is actually worse than worthless because it tends to imply that the clinician made a decision to send the patient home based on information that he should have known was of questionable value.

Once the physician includes acute coronary syndrome in the differential diagnosis—which the ordering of a troponin test indicates—he or she is committed to follow-though. If a decision is made to send a patient home after a single troponin test, the emergency physician should clearly document why this action was appropriate on the basis of timing or the lack of suspicion based on other factors. Indeed, in many busy emergency departments, nurses have ordered a troponin test even before the physician has evaluated the patient. This step should not commit the patient to a full work-up if it is not necessary. But in such cases the wise emergency physician makes a brief mention of why the troponin test was not a relevant factor.

If the troponin level is a relevant factor but has not had time to rise, serial levels are warranted. The physician in this case stated that he did think of serial levels because everything else seemed to point away from a coronary syndrome. He did not document his reasoning, however.

Teaching Points

1. Unless the timing of the test is correct, do not rely on a single troponin level to rule out a myocardial infarction in the emergency department. Even then, unstable angina is not addressed by cardiac enzyme studies in general.

2. If you send a patient home after a single troponin level, make sure to explain your clinical reasoning in the chart. If your reasons were valid but not recorded, they will be assumed not to have existed.

Case 25
Writing on the Wall

A 51-year-old man was brought to the emergency department by his wife after an episode of left shoulder discomfort and "chest weakness," along with some nausea. The episode had occurred earlier that morning and by the time of admission had abated completely. The patient had come only at the insistence of his spouse. The triage note mentioned that the patient was anxious and depressed, having lost his job the previous week.

The emergency physician evaluated the patient, whose vital signs were normal. He said that the sensations in his chest and shoulder were not really pains. He had no diaphoresis, cough, or other symptoms, and had come only to satisfy his wife. He thought that his symptoms were really nothing. The man's wife had left briefly, and the emergency physician did not have the opportunity to speak with her. The man had no known history of cardiac disease, although his father had died in his early sixties from a myocardial infarction. The patient had quit smoking a year or so ago and now exercised regularly, although the loss of his job meant that he might have to stop going to the gym. He had a history of mild hypertension and had briefly taken metoprolol, which was discontinued 6 months ago by his primary physician. He had not slept well for the past 3 nights.

On examination the emergency physician noted that the patient was a little overweight and appeared anxious and fatigued. The exam, however, was otherwise normal. The physician ordered a full set of lab tests, including an EKG, chest x-ray, and troponin level. The EKG appeared to be completely normal, as was the x-ray. The blood work was unremarkable except for a serum glucose of 190 mg/dl. At the end of an approximate 3-hour stay in the emergency department, the patient had remained free of symptoms and wanted to go home. The emergency physician believed that discharge was reasonable. When the man asked for something to help him sleep, the physician prescribed several alprazolam tables and instructed the man to see his primary physician for a good general check-up as soon as possible and to come back if any symptoms returned.

At 7 AM the next morning the patient was brought to the department in full cardiac arrest and did not respond to resuscitation efforts. Autopsy showed severe coronary artery disease and possible signs of an acute myocardial infarction. On review of the case, it became apparent that there were two EKG's in the chart, one of which was normal and belonged to a different patient. The patient's EKG showed unequivocal elevation of the ST segments in V4–V6. A technician apparently had placed another patient's EKG in the chart, and the physician had interpreted the wrong EKG, despite the fact that a different name was clearly printed on it.

A lawsuit was subsequently settled on behalf of the patient's estate.

Analysis

As long as emergency departments become chaotic from time to time, emergency physicians will be at risk for making similar mistakes. When faced with a desk full of lab reports, charts, and EKGs—or, for that matter, a view box full of x-rays to be read—it is only a matter of time before Murphy's law asserts itself, unless scrupulous care is taken to match names to studies. Emergency physicians must habitually check the name on EKGs, lab results, and x-rays.

Reviewers also pointed out that a case for admitting this patient could have been made on the basis of his history and risk factors alone, and that the normal troponin level was of questionable value because it was drawn approximately 5 hours after the onset of chest pain— perhaps too early to have begun rising.

It also became clear that if the emergency physician had spoken with the patient's wife, his level of suspicion for a cardiac problem would have been higher. She had observed the patient that morning sitting on the couch, rubbing his chest, short of breath, and sweating profusely. The patient had been in denial.

Teaching Points

1. Check the name on an EKG, lab slip, or x-ray as part of the reading.

2. Emergency departments should develop systems to minimize the chance that one patient's results end up in the wrong chart.

3. Never place great reliance on a single cardiac enzyme value.

4. Give risk factors great weight in considering a cardiac diagnosis.

5. Whenever possible, speak to people who saw the patient having symptoms. Many patients minimize how bad they feel.

Case 26
Taking Everything to Heart

A 19-year-old Hispanic man first presented to the emergency department on April 9, complaining of chest pains and numbness of his left arm. He spoke no English, but between the emergency physician's rudimentary Spanish and the patient's brother, the emergency physician felt that an adequate history was obtained. The pain appeared to be pleuritic, not associated with chest wall tenderness or auscultatory changes, and had been ongoing for about 24 hours. Vital signs, including pulse oximetry, were generally unremarkable, although the patient's pulse rate was 105 beats/min. The patient was visibly anxious. The emergency physician ordered a chest x-ray, which was read as negative by the radiologist. He gave the patient a dose of ibuprofen and discharged him with the diagnosis of possible pleurisy. No further lab tests were deemed necessary.

On April 10 the patient returned with the same complaint of chest pain. A second emergency physician, who knew no Spanish whatsoever, called for an interpreter and studied the previous day's chart. While still waiting for an interpreter, he examined the young man. Although he was anxious and his skin was slightly sweaty, the patient was afebrile, with normal blood pressure, a heart rate of 105 beats/min, a respiratory rate of 20, and a room air oxygen saturation of 100%. The emergency physician ordered a complete blood count (CBC) and obtained a broken history from the patient's brother, learning that the young man had been previously healthy. Two hours later, the interpreter still not present, the patient's brother asked if they could leave. The emergency physician agreed, discharging him with a diagnosis of anxiety and atypical chest pain. The CBC was normal.

On April 11 the young man again returned with the same complaint. This time the patient's aunt, who spoke excellent English, accompanied him. She was obviously concerned about his discomfort. The patient's vital signs were unchanged from the previous day. His exam remained unremarkable, according to the physician's note. The emergency physician ordered an EKG, which showed only a sinus tachycardia and changes consistent with early repolarization. He also ordered a repeat chest x-ray, which showed no signs of infiltrate or pneumothorax.

The third physician, however, was impressed by the patient's degree of anxiety. The young man seemed to have trouble sitting still on the stretcher. The aunt revealed that the patient's father, who lived in Puerto Rico, had terminal cancer and was expected to die soon and that the young man could not afford a trip home. The emergency physician gave the patient a prescription for 0.5 mg lorazepam tablets and discharged him.

That evening the patient returned. The emergency physician who had seen him initially was again on duty. He reviewed the previous charts and took the patient's aunt aside. He told her that the patient was far too young to have heart problems, that they were running up substantial bills, and that they needed to follow up with a primary physician, as previously instructed. The aunt told the emergency physician that they had tried to make an appointment but could not be seen for over a week. The emergency physician handed her the name of an alternate physician, gave the patient a cursory exam, and discharged him.

Three days later, an emergency department director from a different hospital called the director of the first hospital. He informed him that the young man had been admitted with a diagnosis of viral myocarditis and was quite ill. He asked how it was possible the patient had been to his emergency department four times with no suspicion of the diagnosis.

Analysis

The return-visit patient with nonspecific complaints presents a frustrating situation. Return visits may be related to issues of noncompliance with discharge instructions—the failure of patients, for example, to see the physician to whom they were referred (although, to be fair, this is often due to the difficultly of getting into many primary care physician's offices—even those on the follow-up roster who are obligated to see unassigned patients). In any case, return visits to the emergency department present a golden opportunity to pick up conditions that were missed or not apparent on earlier visits.

Unfortunately, once this patient was labeled as having an anxiety problem, subsequent examiners may have too readily accepted this all-encompassing explanation—not that it may have been easy at any point to make an early diagnosis of myocarditis. The evaluations performed by the first three emergency physicians were reasonable.

During the patient's fourth and final visit to the emergency department, however, the emergency physician allowed frustration to overcome his better judgment. The issue of the patient "running up" excessive bills simply had no place in the discussion. A patient's condition must always remain the primary focus. The evaluation that he then performed was probably too cursory to detect subtle but significant findings that may have pointed to the clinical problem. The language barrier probably did not help matters.

With each subsequent visit, a patient should be given more attention. The emergency physician would be wise to assume that previous examiners missed something until proved otherwise. The emergency physician should approach the situation from a fresh perspective, with a high dose of suspicion that something bad may be hiding in the bushes. When a patient returns for the second or third time in a brief period and no clear diagnosis presents itself, the emergency physician should arrange for further evaluation. In some cases, this may involve consideration of admission; in other instances, the emergency physician may need to arrange definite follow-up personally. Make sure that patients at least have an appointment and know when to go. If nothing else, it spares the patient another emergency department visit and may turn out to save the day.

Teaching Points

1. Avoid becoming frustrated with return-visit patients. Think of the boy who cried wolf.

2. Approach return-visit patients with a fresh perspective and assume that something may have been missed.

3. Be especially vigilant when there is a language barrier between you and the patient.

4. At the end of a second repeat visit for an undiagnosed or vague complaint, the patient should leave with explicit follow-up instructions or be admitted if the case warrants.

Case 27
School Daze

A 16-year-old girl got into a fight with another girl, during the course of which she struck her head on a doorjamb. She was transported to the emergency department by ambulance and on arrival complained of a headache. En route to the emergency department she vomited once but afterward reported no more nausea. The emergency physician examined her. He found a mushy subgaleal hematoma over the occiput but no focal neurologic deficits or other positive finds on exam. The patient said she was thirsty. She drank some cola brought into the room by her mother and then ambulated to the bathroom without apparent difficulty. But she was still complaining of significant headache. The emergency physician ordered 60 mg of ketorolac intramuscularly.

After another hour of observation, during which the headache diminished considerably, the emergency physician discharged her in the company of her mother and gave them standard head injury instructions.

The next morning the mother returned with her daughter. Although the girl had slept well, she woke with a terrible headache and had vomited three times at home. The second emergency physician recorded that the patient seemed "slightly lethargic." Shortly after his examination, a nurse called him urgently into the treatment room, where the patient had begun to have seizure activity. Intravenous lorazepam controlled the seizure. The patient was taken to radiology for a CT, which showed a small intraparenchymal bleed in the frontal cortex. According to the radiologist, it was a classic contrecoup injury.

The emergency physician arranged transfer to the tertiary care center for neurosurgical evaluation. Although the patient did not require surgery and ultimately did well, her mother called the hospital administrator to complain that her daughter's injury had been missed during the first visit.

Analysis

To some extent, the jury is still out about the issue of who needs or does not need a CT after minor head injury. This is often a quandary for cost-sensitive emergency physicians encountering patients who may have suffered a brief loss of consciousness but present to the ED alert, oriented, and without neurologic deficits. A recent multi-center retrospective review from the University of Alberta[1] looked at 1164 cases of pediatric patients with head trauma who had suffered loss of consciousness, amnesia, or disorientation but had no focal deficits or seizures. CT was done in only 171 of these children and was abnormal in 35%—the vast majority of which, however, required no intervention. There were no deaths. The general rate of CT scanning varied tremendously among facilities (from 6% to 26%). The authors concluded that the ATLS text recommendation to order CT scans for all children with head trauma is excessive and that selective CT scanning is reasonable.

A prospective study from Louisiana State University[2] undertook to validate a set of high-risk predictors for intracranial injury in 909 patients with minor head injury, all of whom had suffered a loss of consciousness but had Glasgow Coma Scale scores of 15. The CT was positive for intracranial injury in 6.3% of such patients—but only in those who met at least one of seven criteria: headache, vomiting, any alteration of memory, age above 60, drug or alcohol intoxication, physical evidence of trauma above the clavicles, and seizures. The authors suggest that head CT scans may not be needed for patients with minor head trauma who lack any of these factors.

However, because almost everyone will complain of some degree of headache after a bump on the head, these criteria alone may set the threshold for getting CT too low. But the other criteria certainly seem like reasonable factors for the emergency physician to use in helping to determine who should receive a CT.

In light of these criteria, was there anything about the presentation of the 16-year-old girl that should have triggered the first emergency physician to obtain a CT? He documented that she "had probably not lost consciousness." No witnesses to the injury were there in the emergency department to describe what really happened. The physician later said that he based this statement on the patient's comment that she "wasn't sure" if she had been knocked out.

Loss of consciousness represents a surrogate marker for the degree of force to which the cranium was subjected. Sometimes it can be hard to establish. What is the difference between being knocked out and feeling simply dazed after a blow to the head? Nonetheless, the clinician must attempt to establish whether loss of consciousness truly occurred. The best way is to ask patients if they remember the actual impact. Memory of the impact means that their memory did not lose the ability to process information. But if they cannot remember the impact, the force was great enough to disrupt the memory process. Amnesia for the blow equals loss of consciousness. The greater the force, the longer the amnesia will persist—sometimes for hours, days, or even weeks in proportion to the violence of the injury.

In this case the patient had no memory of the blow to her head. She remembered being in the fight, then being on the floor with people standing around her. The physician had not inquired about her memory of the incident and therefore had a falsely optimistic sense of the situation.

One of the people reviewing the case also raised the question of whether ketorolac—with its potential for the enhancement of bleeding though platelet aggregation inhibition—was contraindicated in this patient. Although no studies measure its potential danger in such situations, physicians obviously should avoid ketorolac, and other nonsteroidal anti-inflammatory drugs in head-injured patients, or any other patient in whom bleeding might be of concern.

Teaching Points

1. Patients who suffered a true loss of consciousness after a head injury are at higher risk of complications.

2. Have a lower threshold for ordering head CTs in patients who lost consciousness after blunt trauma to the head.

3. The best question to ask patients when trying to determine if they lost consciousness is whether they are able to recall the impact.

References

1. Klassen TP, et al: Variation in utilization of computed tomography scanning for the investigation of minor head trauma in children: A Canadian experience. Acad Emerg Med 7:739, 2000.
2. Haydel MJ, et al: Indications for computed tomography in patients with minor head injury. N Engl J Med 343:100, 2000.

Case 28
Upstairs, Downstairs

When an 80-year-old man with a history of dementia did not come back to the house after a routine trip to get the mail, his daughter found him sitting on the sidewalk at the base of his front porch steps with a large abrasion on his forehead and a skin tear on his left arm. Because he was a little unsteady when she tried to help him up, she called 911. He was taken by ambulance to the emergency department.

On arrival, his vital signs were normal and his only complaint was of left shoulder pain and left knee pain. He was able to ambulate unassisted from the medic's gurney to the stretcher. The emergency physician examined him and documented the presence of swelling and abrasion over the left frontal forehead, but the patient denied having any headache and was "at his baseline mental state." He also noted that the patient was not sure why he fell or whether he had been knocked out. Exam also revealed swelling over the left patella, left rib tenderness, and painful movement of the left shoulder. The physician's note further stated that the man's neck exam was completely normal and his neurologic status grossly intact.

The physician ordered x-rays of the chest, pelvis, left hip, and left shoulder—all of which were negative. An EKG and routine labs were also unremarkable.

Because the fall may have been secondary to syncope, the emergency physician called the patient's primary doctor to recommend admission for observation. The primary physician was not particularly receptive to the idea, however, and suggested that they simply keep and observe the patient in the emergency department overnight. The primary physician agreed to see him in the morning. It was already 9 PM, and inpatient beds were tight. The primary doctor would discharge him in the morning if all looked well. The emergency physician concurred and placed the patient in a back room on a telemetry monitor. He then signed out the patient to the oncoming physician at midnight as a case of possible syncope and multiple contusions.

About 1:30 AM, a nurse urgently called the new emergency physician to say that the man had vomited and was "choking on it." The patient was indeed having respiratory difficulty, and it appeared that he may have aspirated. His breathing was stentorous, and his room air oxygen saturation was in the low nineties. The oncoming emergency physician quickly reviewed the chart and ordered a chest x-ray and blood gases. He noted also that the patient was responding sluggishly to questions. The physician asked the nurse about the patient's baseline mentation: was he always this slow to respond? She told him that the man had a history of dementia. Since she had been on duty, he had acted much the same—perhaps a little worse now. She also complained to the physician that the patient did not belong in the emergency department. She did not know "how in the hell" they expected emergency department nurses to do routine neurologic checks, as had been ordered by the first emergency physician, given the small staff.

The emergency physician called the primary doctor and described the aspiration episode. Both agreed that he did not appear to need intubation but would probably develop pneumonitis and definitely required full admission. The primary doctor gave telephone admission orders to the nurse, and the emergency physician returned to seeing new patients. The patient was transported to a step-down unit.

When the primary doctor arrived the next morning, the man had normal vital signs and oxygen saturation. However, he was comatose. A head CT done shortly thereafter revealed a massive subdural hematoma.

After consultation with a neurosurgeon and the patient's family, the patient was placed on comfort care. He expired on the following day. The patient's daughter called hospital administration to ask why the blood clot on her father's brain had not been found while he was still in the emergency department (as the primary physician suggested should have been the case).

Analysis

Reviewers of the case observed that the first emergency physician probably should have been more worried about the possibility of a significant head injury. It had been an unobserved fall, possibly from steps to a concrete sidewalk, with definite external signs of head injury. Of course, such a call is always easy in retrospect. The first physician saw no obvious evidence that a head CT was needed and decided to focus on the possibility that a syncopal episode had caused the fall. He felt that the patient needed inpatient observation, and his decision was appropriate.

The problem began, however, with the decision to keep the patient overnight in the emergency department as a matter of convenience for the admitting physician. There may be a time and place for such accommodation, but we must keep in mind that unless an emergency department has an appropriately staffed area dedicated to observation patients, along with a policy that mandates oncoming physicians to perform a sound reevaluation of observed patients transferred to their care, problems will arise. Unfortunately, the shortage of inpatient beds in recent years, combined with rising emergency department volumes, has made the "boarding" of patients a routine necessity. Patient safety becomes a major concern.

The second emergency physician stated that what he "heard" at sign-out was the report of a patient being observed for syncope overnight in the emergency department because the primary physician had opposed admitting him. When the patient vomited and aspirated, the second physician focused on the respiratory situation. It was not clear to him that the patient's mental status had changed, because he had not examined the patient when he first came on shift.

When patients are transferred to new physicians at shift change time—boarded for whatever reason, or simply in mid-evaluation—wise emergency physicians take nothing for granted and perform a personal reassessment.

Intracranial injury should have remained high in the differential diagnosis for this patient when he vomited and his level of consciousness deteriorated.

Teaching Points

1. Sign-out can be a dangerous time. Physicians faced with the demands of a full load of new patients may assume that all is going as planned with patients transferred to their care from the departing physician. But even under the best of conditions, situations can change for the worst.

2. Avoid, whenever possible, keeping patients whom you feel need to be admitted in the emergency department for the sake of an admitting

physician's convenience. This practice ties up emergency department resources while opening the door to potential error.

3. Exercise worst-case scenario thinking in patients with head injury: any change in mental status, worsening headache, or unexplained vomiting represents an intracranial bleed until proved otherwise.

Case 29
Who Should Read the CT?

A 52-year-old farmer came to the emergency department around noon on a Sunday. He had been working in the hayloft and fell approximately six feet, striking his forehead on a beam. He had a 3-cm laceration near the scalp line. A friend who had been working with him drove him to the emergency department. The day was busy. He was placed in a side room, where he waited approximately 2 hours for the emergency physician to repair the wound. His wife had arrived and was waiting with him. The emergency physician noted that the man had not lost consciousness. He was able to stand and walk into his house after the incident. During the laceration repair, the man began to complain of a severe headache. Reassessment of his neurologic status was normal, but the emergency physician ordered a head CT.

No radiologist was on duty in the hospital on weekends. Special studies such as CTs were sent via the Internet to the radiology department at the hospital's tertiary care affiliate 30 miles away. The turnaround time could amount to hours, depending on the state of equipment and the work load at the city hospital's x-ray department.

Although the CT had been performed and the films developed, the official radiologist's report was still not available an hour and a half later when the man's wife ran out to find a nurse. Her husband vomited and was acting strangely. She also asked the nurse if her husband had told them that he was taking a blood thinner.

The emergency physician promptly broke off from another case to check the head-injured man. His appearance was alarming. He was restless and answered questions sluggishly, and his right pupil appeared slightly larger than his left. The emergency physician, who was not in the habit of looking at CTs because he felt it exceeded the level of his training, immediately placed a personal call to the radiologist in the city, who after several minutes of searching returned with the answer that the patient had a subdural hematoma.

The now comatose patient was intubated and transferred by helicopter to the city. The man recovered but was left with permanent neurologic deficits. The case was brought up for review when the family's attorney called the hospital administrator to discuss settlement.

Analysis

In most cases, emergency physicians train in an environment in which radiologists, or at least radiology residents, are on duty 24 hours 7 days/week. It is therefore possible for a trainee to emerge from a high-quality residency without ever making a decision based solely on his or her own interpretation of any film—CT or plain. Furthermore, many emergency physicians, especially those without the benefit of formal emergency medicine training, feel that there is something sacrosanct about the interpretation of CT and MRI images.

But trepidation about reading CTs, while understandable, is unrealistic and potentially dangerous in the real world, as this case illustrates. Although some conditions, such as subtle subarachnoid bleeding or minimal changes in an unenhanced image of a small brain tumor, certainly require the expertise of a radiographer, emergency physicians must be able to recognize the changes associated with subdural and epidural hematomas. Life-threatening intracranial collections of blood and significant midline shifts are easy to interpret, and are within the bailiwick of all emergency physicians. There is no need to await "official interpretation" in critical situations.

The physician in question readily admitted that he should have checked the CT personally immediately after it was available and would have done so had his index of suspicion been higher. But the man looked in excellent condition when he first arrived. The emergency physician also expressed great surprise in retrospect that the radiology technician, who must have seen the hematoma, had not brought it immediately to his attention. The technician was new and busy, however, and considered her job done when the images were sent off and the films developed.

Furthermore, no one at this time knew the patient was taking warfarin for valvular heart disease. No one had taken a medication history, and the patient had not volunteered the information.

How careful must we be with head-injured patients who are anticoagulated? The risk of relatively minor intracranial damage translating into more significant bleeds does appear to be higher for anticoagulated patients.[1] This caveat should not be taken to mean that every person taking warfarin who bangs his or her head automatically buys a head CT—but caution demands that emergency physicians consider altering their threshold for ordering a CT scan when the situation warrants.

Teaching Points

1. Routinely ask all patients with head injury—no matter how minor—whether they are taking anticoagulants.

2. Head-injured patients taking anticoagulants bear a higher risk that otherwise insignificant intracranial bruises will become more serious. They at least should be observed more carefully.

3. Emergency physicians must be able to interpret the basic life-threatening changes seen on CT scans of the head.

References

1. Li J, et al: Mild head injury, anticoagulants and risk of intracranial injury. Lancet 377:771, 2001.

Case 30
Heading My Way?

The attorney son of an 82-year-old woman called the president of the hospital board to complain that one of his emergency physicians had missed the diagnosis of a blood clot on his mother's brain. She was now in the medical center about to be operated on by a neurosurgeon. She had been a patient in the emergency department a month previously when, while visiting a hospitalized friend, she had stumbled in a hallway and hit her head. She was taken to the emergency department, but, according to the son, the doctor discharged her without x-rays. Four weeks later, when she visited her family doctor because of a worsening headache, the problem was found. CT scan diagnosed a subdural hematoma. They were sure that it resulted from the fall a month ago and could easily have killed her. The board president called the emergency department medical director, asking for a review of the case.

The director reported that he breathed more easily after reading the chart. The patient had been seen in the emergency department by one of the group's best documenters. The chart gave a clear picture of when and how the patient arrived. The fall had been caused by a brief sense of imbalance when the patient turned a corner in the corridor, and such sensations in similar circumstances were common for her. All this was well noted in the record. She did not faint and did not lose consciousness when she hit her head. Her neck was not at all sore, stiff, or tender. She was not taking any anticoagulation medications and, while in the emergency department, developed no significant new symptoms, such as worsening headache, dizziness, visual changes, or chest pain. She ambulated normally, had normal vital signs and a normal neurologic exam, and appeared in no distress. The physician had discharged with definite, specific observation and follow-up instructions.

All of this information was written concisely and legibly on the emergency department chart. The director called both the board president and the patient's son and described in detail why the emergency physician's evaluation was appropriate. Both were satisfied, and the complaint went no further.

83

Analysis

This case clearly proves the beauty of good documentation. The chart showed unequivocally that the emergency physician had done everything in his power to evaluate the patient properly. He addressed the concern of why the patient fell in the first place. Because it had not been secondary to a syncopal episode, no lab work or EKG was indicated. He then noted clearly that the patient had no loss of consciousness or other unusual risk factors for an intracranial injury, such as taking an anticoagulant, and furthermore reported that she had no current symptoms, such as headache or nausea, that raise the stakes. He then described her current physical status, including the normal exam, and even mentioned her ability to ambulate without difficulty. He specifically noted that during her hour-long stay in the emergency department her status did not change.

A head CT at that point was simply not indicated by any current medical standards.

Teaching Points

1. Good documentation involves an understanding of the worst-case scenario and sets forth the major factors underlying the clinician's decision-making.

2. Patients, risk management officers, and juries do not expect physicians to be perfect—only to make reasonable, medically informed decisions in the best interest of those under their care. Never forget that the chart is a real-time forum for displaying this decision-making.

Case 31
The Value of Peer Review

In a certain emergency department, physicians had instituted a peer review system in which every fourth chart, along with codes, transfers, and AMA cases, is reviewed within the next 24 hours by the oncoming physician, who ranks various aspects of care quality and charting on a review instrument. On the first day the system went into operation, the physician on duty came across a chart from the previous day, which outlined the following situation:

A 29-year-old woman came to the emergency department complaining of headache. The physician wrote that the headache had started suddenly while the patient was taking a shower and that she had no previous history of headaches. The headache was not as severe on presentation to the emergency department as it had been initially, when it had been "terrible." The emergency physician wrote that the patient appeared comfortable and that her neurologic examination was within normal limits. Her neck was supple, and she was afebrile. She was given a dose of acetaminophen with codeine and discharged with a diagnosis of "acute cephalgia."

The physician peer-reviewer said that a chill went up her spine when she read the history and saw that nothing further had been done. She called the patient and explained that it may be valuable for her to return for a recheck. The patient, whose headache had subsided almost completely, returned that afternoon. A head CT was normal. The emergency physician performed a spinal tap, finding an abnormal number of red blood cells and slight xanthochromia. The emergency physician arranged for the patient to be transferred to the closest medical center, where an anterior communicating artery aneurysm was clipped on the following day. The patient did well.

Analysis

Although one-fourth or more of patients with subarachnoid hemorrhage present to the emergency department comatose or with significant neurologic deficits, the remainder may have only a headache. But it is a special headache. The headache caused by a subarachnoid hemorrhage is typically intense, not well localized, and of an abrupt onset—so abrupt and explosive that patients often can tell you exactly what they were doing when it started. Many also report that it is unprecedented—the worst headache they ever experienced.

Although emergency physicians need to ask whether it was the "worst headache of your life," the quality of onset is of extreme importance. If, as in the patient described above, the cephalgia began suddenly and severely, a search for subarachnoid hemorrhage must be undertaken. The search begins with a CT. The current standard of care is to perform a lumbar puncture if the CT is negative, for CT may miss as many as 10% of bleeds.

The physician who initially saw the patient was a per-diem moonlighter with an internal medicine background who was relatively new to emergency medicine. Although his training certainly included the evaluation of patients for possible subarachnoid hemorrhages, his office practice had not prepared him for the worst-case scenario thinking that an emergency physician needs to use continuously. He later said that with the patient sitting in front of him looking comfortable and fine, he did not entertain much concern for the possibility of a vascular event. He engaged, so to speak, in best-case scenario thinking.

The physician was required to make a presentation to the group on the evaluation of headaches and was encouraged to attend an emergency medicine board review course.

This case also suggests that peer review systems can have value beyond the mere collection of retrospective data for institutional quality-assurance purposes.

Teaching Points

1. Patients with headache must be asked about the quality of onset of pain as well as its relative severity.

2. Because the headache of a subarachnoid hemorrhage reaches maximal intensity soon after onset, in small bleeds the pain may be fading when you see the patient.

3. In patients suspected of having a subarachnoid headache, if the CT is negative, consideration must be given to the performance of a lumbar puncture.

Case 32
A Matter of Timing

A previously healthy 69-year-old woman presented to the emergency department at 6 AM with the chief complaint of right shoulder and arm pain for the past several days. The record shows, however, that she had a conglomeration of symptoms, including a headache that worsened when she bent forward and an unusual discomfort in the back of both thighs. The symptoms had been present for 3 to 4 four days, but during this time she had experienced no fever, chills, nausea, or other flu-like symptoms. At the end of the history, the physician wrote that friends of the patient worried that she "might be having a stroke." Her vital signs were normal, and her examination was unremarkable. The emergency physician decided that lab testing was not in order. He reassured her that she was not having a stroke and discharged her with the diagnosis of "transient arthralgias."

Three days later the patient returned with a somewhat different chief complaint. The pain in both posterior thighs had continued, but now there was an aching sensation in the low back. The headache was still present when she bent forward, but review of systems remained negative for fever, chills, or other flu-like symptoms. The second emergency physician, clearly puzzled by the range of symptoms, worried about a lumbar problem of some sort and ordered x-rays of the lumbosacral spine, which were negative. A dose of ibuprofen in the emergency department seemed to help. The physician also ordered a complete blood count and chemistry panel, which were normal. The second discharge diagnosis was "possible lumbar disc disease and flu-like syndrome."

Three evenings later—feeling no better—the patient went to a different emergency department, staffed by the same physician group. The same symptoms were present, but family concern had become quite pronounced. Part of the family's frustration seemed related to the patient's minimizing of the situation.

The third emergency physician felt no less puzzled than his two colleagues. The family quickly let him know that in their opinion the patient had not been thoroughly evaluated. Despite having to contend with a busy emergency department, the physician reported that he had no choice but to pull up a chair, sit down, and walk the patient carefully though the entire history of the problem.

On doing so, a disturbing picture came into focus. The actual onset of symptoms was as follows. The patient was sitting at a church meeting when a sudden and strange tingling sort of pain moved up both thighs and, over a minute or so, sped up her back and into her head. When the sensation reached her head, she stated that it felt like "my head was going to explode." Nothing like this had happened to her before. She nearly fainted from the pain. But because she did not want to bother anybody or embarrass herself, she waited it out. After 5 or 10 minutes, the headache and other sensations calmed down. She never mentioned it to anyone, not even her husband, until the meeting was over. For the next few days, she felt like she had been "run over by a truck". Several days later she visited the emergency department for the first time.

The physician performed a thorough examination, including a complete neurologic exam, which was normal. But, concerned by the patient's description of an "explosive" event, he phoned a neurosurgeon in the city, who concurred that the patient may have experienced a central nervous system vascular accident—perhaps spinal. The neurosurgeon accepted the patient for transfer that evening to the medical center.

A strange course followed. An MRI of the spine revealed no abnormalities. While on the table being prepared for a cerebral angiogram, the patient abruptly developed a severe headache and obtundation. Immediate CT revealed a large hemorrhage. After stabilization, she was taken back to the angiography suite, where an aneurysm on the anterior communicating artery was "coiled."

Fortunately, the patient did well, recovering with nearly complete function over the next several months. A family member called the hospital administrator, however, concerned about the initial delay in diagnosis.

Analysis

In retrospect, the patient's initial symptoms obviously came from a "herald bleed"—a minor leakage from an aneurysm preceding a more catastrophic hemorrhage. The extremity symptoms were paresthesias related to cerebral cortical irritation. If the patient had complained of an explosive headache, most emergency physicians would have honed in immediately on the real diagnosis. But she focused elsewhere—and the first two physicians did not peel away enough layers of history and obfuscating symptoms to uncover the true seminal event.

The patient, however, described the headache to a friend—in whose mind the thought of stroke was raised. But it did not occur to the physician to ask the patient why her friend was worried. When patients arrive "prediagnosed" by friends and family members, perhaps sometimes in confusing situations, such impressions can yield clues. The pace of life in the emergency department often feels at odds with the sometimes laborious process of sitting down and burrowing deeply into a puzzling patient's story. But such an effort almost always bears fruit and may save time in the long run.

One reviewer noted that neither of the first two physicians did a thorough job of arranging follow-up. Neither specifically instructed the patient to see her primary doctor, which seemed a little less than adequately vigilant in light of their own inability to find a convincing diagnosis to explain the symptoms.

Teaching Points

1. When dealing with a complex, confusing clinical picture, take an especially careful history, paying close attention to the onset and evolution of symptoms.

2. Any abrupt onset of neurologic symptoms—headache and/or extremity sensations of pain, paresthesias, or weakness—should raise concern for a central nervous system vascular accident.

3. Sometimes it pays to listen to the lay diagnoses offered by patients or their friends and family.

4. When discharging patients who deserve further evaluation, the emergency physician may want to enhance the likelihood of follow-up by specifying time parameters or by making personal contact with the downstream practitioner to transfer information and firm-up logistics.

Case 33
Document, Document, Document

A 29-year-old-woman collapsed two weeks after child delivery and was found on the floor by her husband when he came home from picking up a Sunday newspaper. Their infant daughter was crying in the bedroom. Within several minutes she was able to sit up, then walk, but she had no recollection of falling. The left side of her face, furthermore, felt numb. Her husband left their baby with his mother and took his wife to the emergency department.

On arrival she was alert and oriented. Her vital signs were normal except for a blood pressure of 171/110 mmHg. The recent pregnancy and delivery (her first) had been uncomplicated. She had no history of stroke or seizure disorder but did have a history of migraines, which had been quiescent since pregnancy. She had no headache today.

In his note, the emergency physician described her as acting slightly lethargic. Neurologic exam revealed equivocal left-sided facial droop and possible mild weakness of the left upper extremity. Her neck was supple. There were no carotid bruits and no signs of trauma. He ordered routine labs, an EKG, and a head CT scan. Everything was normal, including the CT.

The emergency physician called the hospital's neurologist, who was making rounds. He examined the patient and reviewed her CT. He agreed that the CT was negative. By this time, the facial droop and arm weakness had completely resolved, and the patient was alert. The neurologist said that a transient ischemic attack (TIA) was possible. He recommended aspirin, and (according to the emergency physician's later recollection) said it would be fine to send the patient home and arrange further work-up, including Doppler carotid studies, on an outpatient basis.

The emergency physician called the patient's internist and reviewed the case. The internist disagreed with the diagnosis of a TIA. He thought that the patient had probably experienced an atypical migraine. The internist told the emergency physician to send her home and have her see him the next morning.

That night, however, the patient had a seizure. Her husband called emergency medical services but wanted his wife taken to a more

distant medical center, where CT scan now showed a cerebral infarction. The patient was admitted and recovered with minor neurologic
deficits.

A hospital administrator at the medical center called her counterpart at
the first hospital and suggested that someone may have dropped the
ball. A thorough review ensued, and it was quickly discovered that the
neurologist's dictated consultation note contained a recommendation to
admit the patient—utterly contradicting the emergency physician's
recollection. The neurologist had dictated this note shortly after seeing
the patient. The best that could be determined was that the emergency
physician may have misunderstood. He continued to maintain that the
neurologist said, "Send her home." The patient's internist joined the
debate and stated that he would definitely have admitted the patient if
he had known of the neurologist's recommendation.

Unfortunately, the emergency physician's note was extremely brief and
made no mention of the neurologist's recommendations. It lacked
even a minimal discussion of clinical reasoning and did not mention
the patient's status at the time of the discharge.

Despite the fact that it probably would have made absolutely no clinical difference whether or not the patient had been admitted, the emergency physician received a letter of reprimand from the executive
committee of the medical staff and was placed on 6 month's probation.

Analysis

The quality and quantity of documentation by emergency physicians
still varies significantly across the country. At one extreme we have
fully dictated notes that rival admission history and physical exams in
their completeness and depth of detail. But many—probably most—
emergency physicians still rely on handwritten notes that range from
the terse to the verbose, and may or may not be legible. A growing
number of emergency departments use template charts, especially
designed with coders in mind, not downstream physicians who have
to read them.

Regardless of chart format, one thing is constant: the best practice is
to describe in one fashion or another your clinical reasoning. This
information tends to flow out naturally in dictated records but is seen
less often in handwritten and template charts. Why is this? Does it
take that much longer to write a few extra sentences than to dictate

them? Or perhaps the informal nature of a handwritten note makes it seem acceptable to omit information.

The goal of the thousands of physicians who still create records by hand should be to make their charts read as much like a dictated chart as possible, with as much legibility as they can muster, and to lay on the detail when it is needed. Detail is most needed in the clinical reasoning and assessment parts of the chart, which also should contain a mention of how the patient did during the emergency department stay. In this way, the emergency physician will have a chart that is maximally useful to the next physician as well as to him- or herself, if a risk-management question arises.

Was it wise for the emergency physician to send the patient home? She had had a syncopal spell by history, followed by apparent neurologic deficits. Given the potential for postpartum hypercoagulability, she was at some risk for more serious episodes. And, more basically, had she experienced a seizure or syncope? And if it was syncope, may it have been cardiogenic? All in all, the more one thinks about the case, the more reasonable it seems simply to have admitted her for observation and evaluation.

Many emergency physicians would have been uncomfortable letting this patient go home—even if both consultant and primary doctor felt it was safe to discharge her.

Teaching Points

1. Pregnancy and postpartum states involve higher risk for thromboembolic disorders.

2. Unexplained acute neurologic symptoms are vascular until proved otherwise.

3. Suggestions by consultants and admitting physicians must be weighed against the emergency physician's own judgment. The liability will rest with the emergency physician at the end of the day.

4. Always document your clinical impression and include a discussion of your diagnostic reasoning. Shoot for making your handwritten final impression and disposition section as complete as you would if it were dictated.

5. Guard yourself against "memory lapses" on the part of consultants by jotting down their recommendations.

Case 34
A Question of Aggression

A 75-year-old man came to a small community hospital emergency department approximately 1 hour after the onset of aphasia, accompanied by a right facial droop and marked weakness of the right arm and leg. His medical history was significant only for hypertension and smoking. He was not diabetic and had no history of a seizure disorder. On arrival at the emergency department he was awake but confused and had great difficulty in forming words. His vital signs were normal except for a blood pressure of 160/97 mmHg.

The emergency physician ordered routine lab tests and a CT, which was read as negative by the radiologist. While studies were pending, the physician questioned the man and his family about possible contraindications to fibrinolytic therapy, which he discussed as a possible option. They appeared to be in agreement.

Once all the lab tests were back, the CT was read, and the exclusion and inclusion criteria were reviewed, the emergency physician and the patient's internist (who came to evaluate the patient in the emergency department) decided to administer tissue plasminogen activator (tPA). The patient signed the consent, with the family as witnesses. He also reconfirmed a standing do-not-resuscitate (DNR) order.

After the tPA was administered, the patient was taken to a general medical floor and over the next several hours rapidly deteriorated. Three days later he died. A repeat CT scan had not been performed.

This was the first time that tPA had been given for stroke in this hospital, and it caused quite a stir—especially because the patient worsened and succumbed. Vigorous criticisms were leveled at the emergency physician and the internist—especially from nursing management. Why had the patient been admitted to a general floor and not the ICU? Why had no repeat CT been ordered? Why, in fact, had the patient not been initially transferred to a tertiary care center, where the services of a neurologist, neurosurgeon, and stroke team would have been available?

This community hospital instituted a moratorium on the use of tPA in stroke patients.

Analysis

Despite approval by the Food and Drug Administration and the American Heart Association's incorporation of tPA for stroke in its ACLS curriculum, there remains a major debate over its actual safety and efficacy.[1-7] Recent articles clearly suggest that, unless selection criteria are rigidly followed, the use of tPA for stroke in community hospitals can lead to significantly worse-than-expected outcomes.[8,9] Given this debate, no clinician should feel compelled by public pressure or fears of medicolegal risk to use tPA in stroke unless they personally believe that it is justified in general and indicated for a particular patient.

Community hospitals that desire to use tPA in stroke patients should approach the issue prospectively though the development of protocols that mandate careful adherence to selection criteria. Emergency physicians, primary care providers, neurologists, and—importantly—nurses should be involved in the creation of such protocols. They can include pathways that indicate the level of required monitoring and contain tools to give nursing staff—who will see such patients infrequently—a simple way to follow and document such aspects as the patient's neurologic status.

The debate over tPA in stroke will continue for a long time, and this treatment modality may gradually slip out of the mainstream into a more limited niche. In the meantime, it remains a matter of individual clinical judgment. Safe use in the community hospital setting requires adoption of protocols and strict adherence to National Institute of Neurological Disorders and Stroke selection criteria.

The emergency physician in this case followed the selection criteria, and if you believe in the value of tPA for stroke, the patient was a reasonable candidate. The decision to admit him to a floor instead of the ICU was based on the fact that the family had a previously existing and subsequently confirmed DNR order. They wanted nothing done if he deteriorated. The furor that followed was largely due to the facility's lack of preparation in general and nursing discomfort specifically—issues that must not be lightly dismissed.

Teaching Points

1. The ultimate value and safety of tPA for stroke patients is still debated.

2. Emergency physicians should not be pressured by reports in the popular media into using tPA for stroke if they believe that it is not clinically warranted.

3. The major problems encountered with the use of tPA for stroke in community hospitals involve failure to adhere to strict inclusion criteria.

4. Community hospitals should have protocols for using tPA in stroke that involve input of nursing and medical staff.

References

1. Hoffman JR: Tissue plasminogen activator for acute ischemic stroke: Is the CAEP position statement too negative? Can J Emerg Med 3(3):183, 2001.
2. Thrombolytic therapy for acute ischemic stroke. Canadian Association of Emergency Physicians Committee on Thrombolytic Therapy for Acute Ischemic Stroke: Can J Emerg Med 3:8, 2001.
3. Lopez-Yunez AM, et al: Protocol violations in community-based rTPA stroke treatment are associated with symptomatic intracerebral hemorrhage. Stroke 32:12, 2001.
4. Tanne D, et al: Initial clinical experience with IV tissue plasminogen activator for acute ischemic stroke: A multicenter survey. Neurology 53:424, 1999.
5. Caplan LR: Stroke thrombolysis: Growing pains. Mayo Clin Proc 72:1090, 1997.
6. Riggs JE: Tissue-type plasminogen activator should not be used in acute ischemic stroke. Arch Fam Med 6(7):102, 1997.
7. Hoffman JR: Should physicians give tPA to patients with acute ischemic stroke? Against: And just what is the emperor of stroke wearing? West J Med 173:149, 2000.
8. Katzan IL, et al: The use of tissue-type plasminogen activator for acute ischemic stroke: The Cleveland area experience. JAMA 283:1151, 2000.
9. Lopez-Yunez AM, et al: protocol violations in community-based rTPA stroke treatment are associated with symptomatic intracerebral hemorrhage Stroke 32:12, 2001.

Chapter Seven

Case 35
The Overdiagnosed Abortion

A 30-year-old pregnant woman came to the emergency department of a community hospital with a history of several hours of vaginal bleeding and lower abdominal cramping. The patient's pregnancy had been confirmed as intrauterine the week before, and the ultrasound showed a gestational age of 7 weeks. It happened to be late on the evening of a major national holiday. The hospital did not have around-the-clock ultrasound availability, and the physician was nearing the final stretch of a 24-hour shift.

The emergency physician performed a pelvic examination and noted, along with a small amount of blood in the vaginal vault, what he believed were obvious products of conception, including an embryo and partial yolk sac. The cervical os was closed. This material was removed and sent for pathologic exam, and a fetal death certificate was filled out.

The patient's bleeding had ceased, and she was in no further pain. The emergency physician diagnosed a completed abortion, contacted her on-call obstetrician, and started the patient on methergine. He then discharged her to follow-up in 2 to 3 days with the obstetrician. The patient filled the prescription and took the medication as ordered.

By the time of the patient's follow-up visit two days later, however, the pathology report was available. The pathologist had seen no products of conception, only decidual uterine material in the specimen. The obstetrician performed an ultrasound, which revealed a viable intrauterine fetus with good fetal heart activity.

The patient and her husband called the emergency department director to complain. They were particularly concerned that the medication prescribed by the emergency physician may harm the fetus.

Analysis

This case amply demonstrates the fact that visual identification of early gestational material can be unreliable. This principle applies to seasoned obstetricians as well as emergency physicians who may only be called upon infrequently to make such a judgment. The diagnosis of completed abortion, therefore, should be withheld unless an undeniably obvious fetal shape is seen or an ultrasound is performed. Furthermore, if any doubt remains after the visual exam of possible products of conception and ultrasound is not available, the emergency physician should avoid prescribing a uterotonic agent, such as methergine. It is questionable, unless significant hemorrhage is occurring, whether a uterotonic agent is needed in the case of a completed abortion.

Should the physician have called in the ultrasound technician from home? Certainly, if there were suspicion of an ectopic gestation, an ultrasound would have been mandatory. If an ectopic pregnancy is a significant consideration and no technician is available, the emergency physician should consider transferring the patient to another facility or, if the patient were highly stable, of observing the patient until an ultrasound could be obtained.

But this patient already had been demonstrated by ultrasound to have an intrauterine gestation. The question was whether she had a threatened, an incomplete, or a completed abortion. In general, it is reasonable to consider performing an ultrasound after every case of possible incomplete abortion. In this case, with an otherwise stable patient, the ultrasound could have been postponed until later that morning—and the methergine withheld.

The patient arrived toward the end of a 24-hour shift. Might this have played a role? The physician was boarded in emergency medicine with over a decade of experience. He admitted not liking 24-hour shifts but did them on occasion to help out. Emergency medicine practice by its very nature sometimes requires "shooting from the hip." Although the problem varies widely for different individuals, common sense tells us that fatigue must affect a physician's decision-making ability. Like it or not, long shifts will be a part of emergency medicine as long as there is a shortage of qualified physicians. As the long day wears on, emergency physicians should become more conservative in their approach to diagnostic testing and consider lowering their threshold for requesting consultations.

Fortunately, the patient's pregnancy remained uncomplicated. A normal infant was delivered on the appropriate date. If the outcome had been poor and litigation had been initiated, the issue of a 24-hour shift would have elicited, in all likelihood, the opposite of sympathy from a jury.

Teaching Points

1. Do not treat an abortion with a uterotonic agent without ultrasound confirmation of completed abortion or an obstetric consultation.

2. Consider the bad outcomes that may result from your treatment plan, and do all you can to avoid them prophylactially.

3. Be careful of—perhaps even second-guess—aggressive management decisions when they come at the end of a long shift.

Case 36

A Matter of Risk

A 35-year-old woman presented to the emergency department with lower abdominal pain that had waxed and waned for the past two days. The pain was somewhat more prominent on the left. She had no history of major illnesses. She had been pregnant three times, had three children at home, and had undergone tubal ligation several years previously. She denied nausea, vomiting, diarrhea, urinary symptoms, or vaginal bleeding since the abdominal pain had begun. Her menstrual cycle had been irregular for many months. Her last period was several weeks ago, and she was having no vaginal bleeding currently.

On arrival, the patient's vital signs were normal. The emergency physician noted that she had "very slight, non-localized tenderness of the lower abdomen, without rebound or guarding." He ordered a complete blood count, which was normal, and a urine pregnancy test, which was positive. The emergency physician told the patient that she needed a pelvic exam. The patient said that she would prefer to have it done by her family physician, who was female and whom she could see the following day. The emergency physician acquiesced and discharged the patient home with instructions to see the family practitioner the next day.

The patient, however, was unable to obtain a timely appointment with her family doctor. Two evenings later the pain abruptly intensified, and the patient fainted. She was brought by ambulance back to the emergency department, now tachycardic and hypotensive. She was typed and cross-matched, resuscitated with fluids, and sent for an urgent ultrasound, which revealed an ectopic pregnancy with significant free fluid in the pelvis. She was taken to surgery and did well.

The gynecologist involved in her case complained to the hospital quality-assurance committee, stating that the diagnosis should have been made when the patient first came to the emergency department.

Analysis

Women who become pregnant after tubal ligation have a high risk of ectopic pregnancy. Other recognized risk factors for tubal pregnancy include the use of intrauterine devices (IUDs), a history of infertility, and a history of pelvic surgery.[1] But any pregnant women who present to the emergency department with more than just minor abdominal pain, with or without vaginal bleeding—especially if the pain is lateralized or if peritoneal signs or cervical motion tenderness is present—are also more likely to have an ectopic pregnancy.

We cannot afford to miss them. Emergency physicians should have an extremely low threshold for obtaining pelvic ultrasonography in pregnant women who have suspicious pain, have undergone tubal ligation, or have a history of infertility or pelvic surgery.

Emergency physicians who both waive the pelvic exam and fail to obtain an ultrasound in such patients court more than a complaint.

Teaching Points

1. Most women of reproductive age with abdominal pain should undergo pregnancy tests.

2. Tubal ligation, pelvic surgery, IUDs, and infertility are risk factors for ectopic pregnancy.

3. Be aggressive in ruling out ectopic pregnancy when patterns of pain or tenderness or risk factors warrant concern.

References

1. Dart RG, et al: Predictive value of history and physical examination in patients with suspected ectopic pregnancy. Ann Emerg Med 33:283, 1999.

Case 37
Primroses and Urinalyses

A 29-year-old woman came to the emergency department complaining of upper abdominal and mid-back pain, accompanied by nausea. The symptoms had begun a few hours before, and the discomfort was now abating. She was approximately 22 weeks into her second pregnancy, and thus far there had been no complications. Her first pregnancy had gone well, and her general health was good.

The emergency physician examined her. She was afebrile, had a normal pulse and blood pressure, and looked comfortable. Except for mild tenderness across the upper abdomen, the exam was recorded as unremarkable. There was no costovertebral angle tenderness. The physician ordered routine lab tests.

The white blood cell count was slightly elevated and the hemoglobin slightly depressed, but not to a concerning degree. Serum glucose and electrolytes were completely normal. A clean-catch urinalysis, however, showed 15–20 white blood cells, along with a trace of leukesterase, a few red cells, 5–10 squamous epithelial cells, and 1+ bacteria. Nitrites were negative. On the basis of these findings, the emergency physician diagnosed "possible early pyelonephritis" and discharged the patient home with a prescription for cephalexin, 500 mg 2 times/day for 10 days.

At home that night, she experienced a burning epigastric discomfort that waxed and waned and kept her from sleeping. The next morning (Sunday) she returned to the emergency department. A dose of Mylanta seemed to help the epigastric discomfort, and she became asymptomatic. The second emergency physician did not repeat any lab tests and discharged her with the diagnosis of "esophageal reflux of pregnancy." She was told to continue the cephalexin for her urinary tract infection and to take around-the-clock antacids.

The patient was not seen again until 9 days later when she visited her obstetrician. At this time she had worsening upper abdominal pain combined with two days of anorexia, diarrhea, and low-grade fever. The obstetrician admitted her for evaluation and treatment of dehydration. Several gallstones were discovered on ultrasound, and a stool sample came back positive for *Clostridium difficile* antigen. The patient spent a week in hospital and was treated with Flagyl for presumed iatrogenic pseudomembranous colitis.

Doubting the emergency physician's original diagnosis of urinary tract infection the obstetrician called for the patient's urine culture report. It was negative, showing less than 10,000 colony-forming units of normal gut flora. He then called the emergency department director to complain, stating that unnecessary antibiotic therapy had caused the patient harm.

Fortunately, she recovered uneventfully and delivered a healthy infant at the expected time. She underwent laparoscopic cholycystectomy 7 month after delivery.

Analysis

The diagnosis of urinary tract infection should not be made on shaky evidence, for it may commit patients to unnecessary antibiotics and lead to overlooking of other diagnoses. For this patient, an attack of cholelithiasis probably brought her to the emergency department for the first and possibly a second time.

There are probably very few truly clean-catch urine samples. It usually is not prudent to base the diagnosis on a positive sample if any epithelial cells are present. Their presence indicates that the sample is contaminated. In point of fact, if the emergency physician needs to base a diagnosis on the results of a positive urinalysis, a catheterized specimen should be considered. During medical school and training, many physicians were taught that in elderly women "occult" urinary tract infections can create a whole host of vague systemic symptoms. One can only wonder whether some of those "occult" infections were really "artifacts" and, as a corollary, what problems may have been missed. The emergency physician should not make the same mistakes.

Once the first emergency physician saw the "positive" urinalysis, even though the clinical picture did not fit well at all with an upper urinary tract infection he apparently stopped considering other possibilities.

Teaching Points

1. Never trust positive clean-catch urine specimens when squamous epithelial cells are present—which is almost always.

2. Be especially distrustful when the symptoms do not fit the picture.

3. The risk of missing important diagnoses and committing people to unnecessary medication is at stake.

Case 38
An Ounce of Suspicion

A 19-year-old woman presented to the emergency department one busy afternoon complaining of two days of increasingly painful urination. She had no fever, chills, nausea, vomiting, or flank pain. She was otherwise completely healthy and taking no medications, including birth control. Her last period was approximately 4 weeks ago. On exam she was afebrile and in no acute distress. She had no abdominal or costovertebral angle tenderness. Her urinalysis showed > 25 white blood cells, along with a few red blood cells and epithelial cells. A urine pregnancy test was negative. The emergency physician prescribed sulfamethoxazole-trimethoprim and pyridium and discharged the patient with instructions to take plenty of fluids.

The next day she returned and was seen by another emergency physician in the same department. She had not improved on the medicine. In fact, she now could hardly stand the pain of urination. The second physician checked with the lab to see if culture and sensitivity tests had been ordered the day before. They had not. He told the patient that she probably had a resistant organism and gave her a prescription for ciprofloxacin as well as for acetaminophen with codeine and instructions to try urinating while sitting in a tub of warm water. He also put a copy of the chart in the first emergency physician's mailbox and attached a note asking why a culture had not been ordered.

The patient, unfortunately, returned the next day, her symptoms even worse. It was so painful to urinate that she literally had not done so for the past 7 or 8 hours. She was still afebrile and had no nausea or flank pain. The third emergency physician decided to start from scratch. She pulled up a chair and questioned the patient carefully about her symptoms. She discovered that, although the young woman was experiencing dysuria, she had no urinary urgency or frequency. Moreover, the pain of urination was distinctly external. She told the physician that it felt as if the urine were burning when it hit the outside, as if there were sores around the opening.

The third emergency physician had the patient disrobe, placed her on the pelvic table in stirrups, and examined her external genitalia. She quickly discovered the problem: vesicles, ulceration, and swelling around the labia minora and introitus. One of the lesions was next to the urethral opening.

The emergency physician diagnosed a primary episode of herpes genitalis, which was confirmed by culture. She started the patient on a course of famcyclovir and prescribed viscous xylocaine for pain relief.

Analysis

Women having a primary episode of herpes genitalis may become aware of the condition as a result of painful urination and present to the emergency department with dysuria as the chief complaint. It seems hard to believe, given the presence of lesions and swelling, but this presentation is not uncommon. A clinician who takes dysuria at face value will falsely diagnose the condition as a simple bladder infection. Because the condition is often accompanied by a purulent exudate around the urethra, a clean-catch urine appears positive for pyuria and seems to confirm the diagnosis.

Dysuria, therefore, is a deceptive symptom. To be of diagnostic value, the patient must be asked whether the sensation is internal or external. Many patients cannot clearly differentiate between the two. Far more useful symptoms characteristic of bladder infections are the triad of frequency, urgency, and hesitation. Patients have to urinate badly and often, and little urine is discharged—and yes, a burning sensation is present, but more on the inside. By focusing on this picture, the emergency physician is less likely to be led astray by the complaint of dysuria. If the triad is not present, look for something else to explain the burning sensation—especially lesions on the external genitalia.

The clinician must keep in mind, of course, that pregnancy also can give the sensations of urinary urgency, frequency, and hesitation. The first emergency physician was correct to obtain a pregnancy test. But was he wrong not to culture the urine, as the second emergency physician—who also missed the correct diagnosis—suggested? No. Ample literature demonstrates that urine cultures in healthy, nonpregnant women with only lower tract signs are not cost-effective and should be avoided.

The "positive" urinalysis obtained by the first emergency physician was clearly a contaminated specimen. Squamous epithelial cells were present. Most supposed clean-catch samples contain external material and are not reliable. Patients with herpes simplex virus II (HSV II) infections or vaginitis commonly have contamination pyuria. If squamous epithelial cells are present in the urine in a case in which the results of the urinalysis are of critical importance, a catheterized specimen should be obtained. In a healthy young woman with *all* of the classic symptoms of a bladder infection, however, the results of a urinalysis are almost irrelevant in terms of treatment decisions.

Teaching Points

1. Unless the classic symptoms of urgency, frequency, hesitation, and internal dysuria are present, rule-out an HSV II infection.

2. Do not rely on the results of contaminated urine specimens.

3. Many "clean-catch" urine specimens are contaminated, as evidenced by the presence of squamous epithelial cells.

4. The changes of pregnancy can yield symptoms of urinary urgency, frequency, and hesitation.

Case 39
Stopping Short

A 53-year-old transcontinental truck driver had been experiencing trouble urinating. Despite a strong sense of urgency, for the past 36 hours he had been able to urinate in only small amounts. Because of this and worsening lower abdominal pain, he finally turned off the Interstate at an exit with a hospital sign. He walked into the emergency department at 11 PM, 600 miles from home. According to the triage note, he looked quite uncomfortable.

The man had not experienced a similar problem in the past. Aside from hypertension, for which he was taking atenolol, he had no other medical problems. His vital signs were normal. The emergency physician examined him, noting an occasional expiratory wheeze, no costovertebral angle tenderness, and mild suprapubic tenderness and fullness. He ordered a urinalysis but did not perform a rectal exam.

The man was able to produce about 20 ml of urine, which was sent to the lab and showed 0–2 red blood cells and 10–15 white blood cells per high power field. After ordering a culture of the urine, the emergency physician discharged the patient with ciprofloxacin, acetaminophen with codeine, and a diagnosis of "probable cystitis." He instructed the patient to follow-up with his primary physician.

The patient made his way to a nearby motel but returned to the emergency department 2 hours later because of worsening pain in the lower abdomen. He had been unable to urinate since leaving the emergency department. The same emergency physician was on duty. Reassessing the situation, he decided to place a Foley catheter. Several attempts were unsuccessful, however, and the patient insisted that he stop the attempts. He then urinated an unspecified amount and said that he felt better. The emergency physician discharged him, this time with six Percocet tablets. He instructed the man to visit a urologist as soon as he could.

On the following day, this case drew the attention of the peer reviewer, who wondered why more aggressive efforts to catheterize the patient had not been undertaken on the first visit, when the initial diagnosis of urinary tract infection seemed unsatisfactory. The case was sent to the quality-improvement office and emergency department director for investigation and follow-up. The patient's outcome is unknown. Calls to his home in a different state were not returned. It is very likely that his condition would have led him to seek care at another facility along the way.

Analysis

The patient almost certainly had bladder outlet obstruction secondary to a prostate condition. In men, the diagnosis of isolated cystitis is so uncommon that it should be a diagnosis of exclusion only after urinary retention and prostatitis have been excluded. The emergency physician later said that he considered the diagnosis of prostatitis on the first visit and was not sure why he had written only "cystitis" on the chart. He said that as long as he was going to treat the man with an antibiotic that would cover prostatitis, it seemed reasonable to spare him the discomfort of a rectal exam. Furthermore, he said that the man initially minimized the symptoms suggesting retention, and it became obvious that he could not urinate only on the second visit.

As to the failed catheterization attempts, the emergency physician reported that the man had become hostile and was bleeding from the meatus: "There was no way he was going to let me try again." Moreover, no urologist was on call for the hospital. He believed that his best option was to discharge the patient to make his own follow-up arrangements.

But was it the best option for the patient? It was almost a given that he would need help long before he arrived home. Urinary retention is an extremely painful condition. The patient would be compelled to throw himself at the mercy of yet another emergency department. The quality-improvement committee unanimously believed that the emergency physician should have made contact with the urology service at the local medical center and arranged definitive follow-up, transferring the patient if need be. The emergency physician reported that he did stress the importance of follow-up, but there was no documentation of this claim. There was also no mention that the patient had been told of the potential renal complications that might ensue if the urinary retention was not addressed in a timely fashion.

We are left with the impression that the patient's suffering was his and his alone to deal with as best he could, far from home. The quality-improvement committee was rightly unimpressed by the physician's reasoning behind avoidance of the rectal examination. Prostate cancer, after all, was in the differential diagnosis.

Teaching Points

1. Symptoms of urinary urgency, frequency, and hesitation in men warrant consideration of bladder outflow obstruction. Cystitis in men is a diagnosis of exclusion.

2. A rectal examination must be performed in men with potential prostate disease.

3. In patients with urinary retention in whom catheterization is unsuccessful, on-site consultation or timely follow-up with a urologist is mandatory.

Case 40
You Have to Touch the Patient

A 22-year-old man presented to a busy emergency department with severe pain in the right suprapubic area with radiation to the groin. The pain begun suddenly just after awaking from a nap. The pain was rated as 10 on a scale of 10, and the patient was doubled over. No position was found to make him comfortable. Aside from sinus tachycardia of 110 beats/min, vital signs were normal.

After a brief interview and exam, the emergency physician made the working diagnosis of renal calculus and started the patient on intravenous fluids and pain medications. A urinalysis subsequently showed 1–2 red blood cells with 0–2 white blood cells. The pain, meanwhile, subsided dramatically with pain medication. The emergency physician elected to order an intravenous pyelogram (IVP). The IVP was performed, and the radiologist called the emergency physician to report that it had been negative. There were no obvious signs of obstruction or hydroureter.

By now the pain was minimal. The emergency physician diagnosed a passed kidney stone and prescribed hydrocodone with acetaminophen, telling the patient that additional small stones may pass over the next few days and that he should ride out the pain using the pills unless it became too severe. He also was told to follow up with his primary doctor in 1 week.

The patient indeed continued to have pain at home and used the pain medication as prescribed. One week later he presented for follow-up as instructed. The pain in the groin had localized almost exclusively in the right testicle, which had become swollen and discolored. On performing a complete examination, the primary doctor uncovered and later confirmed by ultrasound the diagnosis of testicular torsion. The testicle could not be salvaged, and there was some question about the viability of the other testicle.

The patient initiated a lawsuit that was successfully settled out of court for a significant sum.

Analysis

Unfair as it may be, emergency physicians are never forgiven for failing to do a thorough examination because of a busy shift. Although it was understandable that the patient's symptoms raised thoughts of a kidney stone, which seemed to be confirmed by the microhematuria found on urinalysis, the emergency physician closed off the differential too early.

Male patients with kidney stones must be questioned thoroughly about the presence of testicular pain, and an examination of the genitalia must be routinely performed if there is any question. Many patients with kidney stones indeed have pain radiating to the testicles, but we must not allow this possibility to lull us into complacency.

The emergency physician actually had a second chance to make the right diagnosis. Ordinarily, even after a stone has passed, for some hours there is some degree of residual hydroureter and hydronephrosis. A completely normal IVP in a patient suspected of kidney stones—especially, as in this case, when any pain remains—should cause the emergency physician to reevaluate the original diagnosis.

Teaching Points

1. Testicular torsion is in the differential diagnosis of patients with potential renal colic. Always exercise worst-case scenario thinking.

2. If the IVP is completely negative, reevaluate the diagnosis of kidney stone.

Case 41
None of Your Beeswax

A 25-year-old woman came to the emergency department two days after being stung by a yellow-jacket on her right forearm, with remarkable swelling and redness nearly to the elbow. She was afebrile and had normal pulse and blood pressure. She had no sign of an allergic reaction elsewhere—no difficulty with breathing or swallowing. No redness and no red streaks were present above the elbow. The patient denied any previous reactions to bee stings and was allergic only to penicillin.

The emergency physician documented the swelling and redness and the otherwise generally negative exam. She prescribed a tapered course of prednisone and a 5-day regimen of cefalexin, discharging the patient with the diagnosis: bee-sting reaction—possible early cellulitis.

The next day the patient developed a hive-like rash on her trunk and went to see her primary physician. The primary physician told the patient that she was having an allergic reaction to the antibiotic and wrote a note to the hospital critical of the emergency physician's decision to prescribe cefalexin when it was both unnecessary and contraindicated by the history of allergy to penicillin.

The patient's swelling and redness resolved within several days, and her hives were gone the day after she stopped taking cefalexin.

Analysis

Patients present to emergency departments after bee stings with one of three syndromes. The most serious and least common is true anaphylaxis. The second and much more frequent scenario is simple urticaria. The third is local tissue swelling around the bite site. This reaction is not an allergic phenomenon and does not produce systemic symptoms, although some patients experience malaise and myalgias. Patients with an isolated local reaction to hymenoptera venom may present a day or two after the sting, often alarmed by the degree of swelling—an entire hand or forearm puffed up and red. They do not appear toxic otherwise.

Some physicians unfamiliar with the local reaction syndrome hedge their bets and put the patient on antibiotics for possible cellulitis. But this strategy is illogical and carries the potential for harm, as the case above demonstrates.

Local reactions to bee venom resolve within 3–7 days, regardless of treatment. Warm compresses, elevation, and reassurance are useful. No definite evidence indicates that steroids or antihistamines speed resolution, although some physicians prescribe these adjuncts empirically.

The primary care physician was correct in stating that the patient did not need antibiotics, but his contention that cefalexin was contraindicated because of the penicillin allergy was inaccurate. We probably do not know the exact incidence of cross-sensitivity between penicillin and the cephalosporins, but common experience holds it to be less than 10%. A recent paper reaffirms this estimate.[1]

A safe rule when contemplating the use of a cephalosporin in a patient with penicillin allergy is first to question the patient about the type of reaction to penicillin. If the patient had an anaphylactic reaction to penicillin, the wisest course is to avoid *parenteral* cephalosporins, if reasonable alternatives are available. If no alternatives are available, consider skin testing before administering the full dose. Most physicians are comfortable giving oral cephalosporins to penicillin-allergic patients, although it is reasonable to inform patients of the small risk and to have them discontinue the medication, take benadryl, and obtain follow-up if any problems arise.

Teaching Points

1. Local reactions to bee stings can resemble cellulitis but should not be treated with antibiotics.

2. Local reactions to bee stings are self-limited. You can treat them effectively with compresses, elevation, and antihistamines if pruritus exists.

References

1. Herbert ME, et al: Medical myth: Ten percent of patients who are allergic to penicillin will have serious reactions if exposed to cephalosporins. West J Med 175:341, 2000

Case 42
Avoiding Medication Mishap

Just as similar cases seem to come to the emergency department in two's and three's, so do errors. In one week two cases involving medication mishaps arose in different patients seen by the same emergency physician.

In the first case, a 45-year-old man with insulin-dependent diabetes, had been ordered 15 units of regular insulin and received 150 units. By the time it was discovered, the patient's glucose had dropped to 50. He was not symptomatic; he was given additional glucose and suffered no further problems. The physician's handwriting was not among the best. His letters tended to be small and steeply slanted, and he frequently used abbreviations. In this case he used a "U" to indicate "units." The error arose when a new nurse interpreted 15U as 150. She was a bit surprised by the amount and went to check her nursing drug handbook, which, interestingly enough, lists doses of regular insulin that were not inconsistent with the one she misinterpreted. She later said that she should have checked with the physician but did not want to "look stupid."

The second case had nothing to do with the physician's handwriting. He had ordered a 5,000-unit bolus of heparin in a patient with thrombophlebitis of the leg. The nurse picked up a vial of the far more concentrated heparin used for flushes, and the patient was administered 40,000 units. This error was discovered by the nurse, who immediately informed the physician. The patient was given protamine sulfate and observed in the ICU for several days. Although the patient developed transient gross hematuria, she ultimately did well without long-term complications.

Analysis

Patient care in the emergency department is and always will be a team effort. Each member of the team must facilitate every other member's ability to function. Physicians who write ambiguous orders hamper the efficiency of nursing personnel who must carry out those orders. Managers who stock pharmacy cabinets with medications of different concentration create an environment in which mistakes are more likely to occur.

Teaching Points

1. Physicians must habitually take great care in writing down orders and avoid unnecessary abbreviations that may lead to misinterpretations.

2. "Units" should be written as such.

3. When micrograms may be confused with milligrams, both terms should be written out fully.

4. When a decimal point precedes a number, a zero should be written before the decimal point.

5. Emergency department directors and nurse managers should review their pharmacies for the presence of medications in different concentrations and create systems that minimize the chance of error.

Case 43
One Man's Poison

A 10-year-old boy came to the emergency department with several deep dog bites to the right ankle. He had no neurovascular deficits on exam. The emergency physician anesthetized the wounds (the largest of which involved a 2-cm wide by 1-cm deep laceration), irrigated with saline, and loosely approximated the edges. The patient was discharged on a 7-day course of ciprofloxacin. He also was given a tetanus booster.

On peer review the case was pulled for further analysis based on the emergency physician's choice of antibiotic and his decision to suture the wounds.

Analysis

The peer reviewer who flagged this chart noted that fluoroquinolones in general are contraindicated in children because of the risk of arthopathy. Is this concern valid? When the fluoroquinolones were first introduced, they carried a contraindication for use in the pediatric population, based on laboratory research that demonstrated joint toxicity in juvenile animals.[1] Subsequent clinical studies in fairly large populations of children seem to suggest, however, that this concern may not be as great as initially feared.[2] Nonetheless, the situation remains somewhat equivocal, and the wisest approach is to reserve the use of fluoroquinolones to brief courses in cases in which no good alternatives exist.

But, pediatric toxicity aside, was ciprofloxacin a good choice bacteriologically? And was antibiotic prophylaxis necessary to begin with?

Currently no hard and fast evidence-based recommendations demand the use of prophylactic antibiotics in dog bites—except when the wound is considered to be at very high risk (i.e., wounds of the hand and patients at high risk due to compromised immune systems). Many clinicians, however, empirically consider any deep dog bite to present a significant risk, especially when the wound involves distal extremities or when the wound is a deep one to the face and has undergone closure with sutures.

Dog-bite infections usually arise from organisms found in the animal's mouth and are often polymicrobial—predominantly alpha-hemolytic streptococci, *Pasteurella multocida*, and *Staphylococcus aureus*. But in up to 40% of such infections anaerobes also are present. The current recommendations for prophylactic antibiotics in high-risk dog bites favor the use of either amoxicillin/clavulanate, a second-generation cephalosporin, or clindamycin plus a fluoroquinolone. These antimicrobials, given for 3–5 days, yield both aerobic and anaerobic coverage.

Although the flora involved in cat-bite infections are somewhat different and the risk of infection somewhat higher, the antimicrobials recommended for prophylaxis are the same as for canine wounds.

Ciprofloxacin, therefore, was not a good choice. Of interest, the physician reported that he understood the recommendations fairly well but choose ciprofloxacin because he had access to samples and knew that the patient's parents had no prescription plan and could not afford to buy an expensive prescription of amoxicillin/clavulanate, the drug of choice.

What about his decision to close the wound? Although it is reasonable and common practice to suture facial lacerations caused by dog bites after thorough cleaning, the risk of infection increases in the extremities, and cosmetic concern decreases. Many authors, therefore, recommend allowing dog bites on the distal extremity to heal by secondary intention. If he had left the wounds open, the need for giving an antibiotic would have been theoretically less.

Calls were placed to the patient's home. The wounds healed well, without complications.

Teaching Points

1. Consider antibiotic prophylaxis in high-risk dog and cat bites, especially those in distal extremities, and immunocompromised patients.

2. The drugs most useful for prophylaxis in dog bites have anaerobic coverage and include amoxicillin/clavulanate, second-generation cephalosporins, and clindamycin plus a fluoroquinolone.

3. Consider allowing dog bites of the extremities to heal by secondary intention.

4. Do *not* base prescription decisions on the presence of free samples. The downstream costs may be much higher.

References

1. Stahlmann R, et al: Quinolones in children: Are concerns over arthropathy justified? Drug Safe 9(6):397, 1993.
2. Kubin R: Safety and efficacy of ciprofloxacin in paediatric patients: Review. Infection 21(6):413, 1993.

Chapter 9
Gastrointestinal Problems

Case 44
Keeping It Down

A 47-year-old woman came to the emergency department after 3 days of diarrhea and vomiting and poor oral intake. She had a history of numerous hospital admissions for severe asthma, which had been quiescent recently. She was taking a steroid and brochodilators by metered-dose inhaler at home, and for the past 6 months she had been taking 20 mg/day of prednisone. She was otherwise healthy.

Her vital signs were normal except for a pulse rate of 115 beats/min, which rose to 130 when she stood by the bedside without a drop in blood pressure. The emergency physician wrote that she was a very slender, tired-looking woman whose oral mucous membranes were dry. Chest auscultation revealed only mild expiratory wheezing. Her bowel sounds were normal, and her abdomen was soft to palpation, without masses or organomegaly.

The emergency physician ordered labs and intravenous normal saline, 2 liters over 2 hours. He also ordered a dose of intravenous promethazine.

The complete blood count was normal. Serum chemistries were also normal, except for a mildly elevated blood urea nitrogen. After the 2 liters of saline the patient said that she felt better. She had no episodes of diarrhea in the emergency department, and the nausea had abated. She was able to tolerate liquids. The emergency physician diagnosed nonspecific gastroenteritis and discharged the patient with a prescription for trimethobenzamide (Tigan) suppositories and instructions to use Peptobismol if the diarrhea returned

Although her diarrhea resolved, over the next two days the patient continued to vomit and was unable to tolerate much of anything by mouth. She was also becoming lethargic and weak. Two days after the first visit, her husband, who had been disappointed that his wife was not admitted to the hospital initially, took her to a different emergency department. At the second hospital she was diagnosed with dehydration and adrenal crisis caused by steroid withdrawal. She had been unable to hold down the prednisone since the onset of her symptoms several days before the first emergency department visit. The emergency physician at the second hospital told the patient and her husband that this problem should have been addressed during the first visit. She was admitted, hydrated, treated with intravenous hydrocortisone, and recovered well.

But her husband called the first hospital to complain, saying that the emergency physician failed to asked his wife about the prednisone and that nothing had been done for her.

Analysis

As a brief refresher: adrenal insufficiency can be caused by a problem anywhere along the hormonal axis, from the hypothalamus to the adrenal glands. *Primary adrenal insufficiency* (Addison's disease) occurs when the adrenal glands are physically compromised by autoimmune, idiopathic, infectious, infiltrative, or hemorrhagic processes. *Secondary adrenal insufficiency* results from a failure of the pituitary gland to produce sufficient quantities of adrenocorticotropic hormone (ACTH). *Tertiary adrenal insufficiency* implies an upstream failure of the hypothalamus to produce enough corticotropin releasing factor (CRF) to regulate the pituitary.

The most common cause of tertiary adrenal dysfunction is the iatrogenic suppression of the entire axis by exogenously administered glucocorticoids, which leads to functional and physical atrophy of the adrenal glands. The sudden withdrawal of exogenous glucocorticoids can be life-threatening.

Addison's disease can be difficult to diagnose in the emergency department. The symptoms and signs are varied and diffuse. It should be suspected in patients with chronic or subacute weakness, lethargy, postural hypotension, anorexia, nausea, diarrhea, and weight loss. Mental status changes may be present. Patients also may show cutaneous manifestations, such as hyperpigmentation of exposed areas and pressure points. And, unlike adrenal insufficiency caused by reduced levels of ACTH (secondary and tertiary adrenal insufficiency), primary adrenal insufficiency is associated with diminished levels of mineralocorticoids. The clinician, therefore, should be alert for electrolyte abnormalities, especially hyponatremia and hyperkalemia, when considering this diagnosis.

But, far and away, the adrenal issue of most concern to emergency physicians is iatrogenic adrenal suppression by exogenous steroids and the crisis that can arise from acute withdrawal. Any patient who has been taking prednisone at a dosage greater than 10–20 mg for more than 3 weeks should be assumed to have adrenal suppression. Even minor illnesses in such patients should make the physician consider a supraphysiologic "stress dose" of steroid. Any question that such a patient may be entering adrenal crisis warrants admission and intravenous glucocorticoids. Begin treatment in the emergency department with 100 mg of hydrocortisone intravenously.

Teaching Points

1. Adrenal suppression begins after 3 weeks of prednisone at dosages of 10–20 mg/day.

2. Be alert when steroid-dependent patients present to the emergency department with gastroenteritis symptoms. Make sure that they have been taking and keeping down their medications.

3. Consider giving stress doses of steroids to any steroid-dependent patient with even a minor illness.

4. Be aggressive when dealing with patients at risk for steroid withdrawal.

Case 45
What's Eating You?

A 75-year old man with non–insulin-dependent diabetes mellitus presented to the emergency department with abdominal pain. The pain was steady and mainly epigastric, but seemed to move toward the mid-back, although the patient could not describe this movement precisely. He also became nauseated and had vomited once before coming to the emergency department. He said that the emesis was dark and maybe a little granular-looking. It was just after the holidays, and he had eaten a lot of his favorite cheese lately. He thought that this explained why he had not had a bowel movement in a few days despite laxatives. His current medications were glipizide, hydrochlorothiazide, occasional ibuprofen for arthritis pain, and one enteric-coated aspirin per day. He had a distant history of peptic ulcer disease but denied similar pain previously.

The emergency physician described the patient as looking uncomfortable but stable. He was afebrile, his blood pressure was 175/95 mm Hg, and his pulse rate was 110 beats/min. The exam was unremarkable except for "nonspecific" epigastric and upper-quadrant tenderness. The rectal exam was negative for occult blood. The physician ordered a nasogastric tube to check the gastric contents for blood. The test was negative. He also ordered a panel of routine lab tests. Meanwhile, the patient's pain was beginning to resolve.

The white blood cell count was 8,700/μl. Hemoglobin and electrolytes were normal, and serum glucose was elevated at 190 mg/dl. A free-air series was negative for free air or abnormal gas patterns, but a lot of stool appeared to be present. The EKG was unchanged from the EKG done a year previously. The emergency physician ordered a dose of intravenous ranitidine and a bottle of magnesium citrate and discharged the patient with a diagnosis of constipation vs. gastroenteritis.

Two days later the same man returned and was seen by a different emergency physician. The magnesium citrate had worked, and the patient no longer felt constipated, but his abdominal pain had returned shortly after trying to eat lunch. It was worse than ever, and he had been vomiting all afternoon. The pain seemed to worsen with respirations, and he had a chill just before coming to the emergency department. He also admitted to having a slight cough and to feeling a little short of breath.

On reexamination, his vital signs were fairly unremarkable. Once again he was afebrile with nonspecific upper abdominal tenderness without guarding or rebound. During the exam the emergency physician noted that he coughed occasionally. She ordered another round of lab tests and x-rays, both a free-air series and a posteroanterior and lateral chest views, and asked the nurse to perform a pulse oximetry measurement, which showed an oxygen saturation of 97% on room air. She ordered an infusion of normal saline at 150 ml/hour and a single intravenous dose of 12.5 mg promethazine for the nausea.

The white blood cell count was 11,700/μl with a slight left shift. Blood sugar was 180 mg/dl. Electrolytes were normal, but the blood urea nitrogen was slightly elevated. A urinalysis was normal, and a repeat EKG was unchanged. On chest x-ray, however, the emergency physician believed that she detected a new, small infiltrate at the base of the right lung.

Meanwhile, the patient's abdominal pain had dissipated and his nausea resolved. The emergency physician asked the nurses to give the patient a trial of clear liquids, and ordered an oral dose of azithromycin. She told the patient's family that the abdominal pain probably was caused by pneumonia. The patient was able to tolerate clear liquids without a problem and was subsequently discharged with the diagnosis of "probable early pneumonia" and a prescription for a full course of azithromycin.

The patient, however, returned the following day. He had vomited throughout the night and had several shaking chills; the pain was even worse. On arrival he appeared weak and dehydrated and, according the physician's note, "borderline septic." His blood pressure was 110/54 mm Hg and his pulse rate 115 beats/min. His oral temperature was normal, but the emergency physician asked the nurse to obtain a rectal temperature because the patient felt warm. The rectal temperature was 102.3° F.

The third emergency physician reviewed the previous two work-ups and discovered that the radiologist had disagreed with the second physician's belief that pneumonia was present. The chest x-ray was read as normal.

On examination, the patient's abdomen now seemed most tender in the right upper quadrant, although there was no guarding or

Murphy's sign. While blood work was pending, the patient was sent for abdominal ultrasound, which showed gallstones and changes consistent with cholecystitis. He was started on intravenous antibiotics and admitted. On subsequent cholecystectomy, the gallbladder was full of pus and becoming necrotic. Although he eventually recovered, the patient's postoperative course was not smooth and included a bout with acute respiratory distress syndrome.

The patient's family filed a formal complaint because he had been sent home twice with the wrong diagnosis.

Analysis

Make no mistake: abdominal pain in elderly patients is one of the scariest presenting complaints that an emergency physician can face. Terrible problems can lurk behind minimal findings, as amply documented in recent papers.[1,2] Clinical findings in elderly patients who present to emergency departments with abdominal pain are far more likely to be nonspecific than in younger people, and age-related memory deficits can make the history less reliable. Many elderly patients also have comorbidities such as diabetes that add to the difficulty of interpreting clinical signs and symptoms because of neuropathic alterations in pain perception. Significant minorities of elderly patients with infections such as cholecystitis, diverticulitis, and appendicitis may present without fever or characteristic physical findings or lab abnormalities.

Given this background, the emergency physician needs to maintain a high index of suspicion in elderly patients with abdominal pain. It may be wise in many cases for the emergency physician to lower his or her threshold for performing comprehensive evaluations (e.g., to order ultrasound more routinely) and to admit ambiguous cases for observation.

The first emergency physician's evaluation was reasonable in most regards, although in retrospect the association of the pain with a recent meal was a clue to the true diagnosis. Certainly, no one would have faulted him for ordering an ultrasound even if it turned out negative. The second emergency physician appeared to have jumped to the diagnosis of pneumonia on insufficient evidence. But there was not enough compelling evidence of intraabdominal pathology—or so it seemed—to move her further in that direction. Pneumonia, on the other hand, did not explain adequately the range of symptoms.

The simple fact of a second, unplanned visit for abdominal pain in an elderly patient—some would say with justification—is grounds for admission and a thorough evaluation for intraabdominal disease.

One more point is worth noting: the unreliability of the oral temperature in this patient. The physician's clinical sense told him that the patient had a fever despite the normal oral temperature. Because the presence of a fever clearly raises the ante in regard to the potential seriousness of abdominal pain in an elderly patient and because the elderly patient may be less able to cooperate with obtaining an oral temperature, a wise practice is to ask for a rectal temperature in any patient for whom the presence of a fever might make a difference in diagnosis and disposition.

Teaching Points

1. The usual signs, symptoms, and laboratory abnormalities associated with abdominal infections may be diminished or absent in elderly patients.

2. Elderly patients with abdominal pain are more likely than younger patients to be hiding something serious. Consider more comprehensive evaluations, and lower your threshold for admitting such patients.

3. Many elderly patients sent home with the diagnosis of constipation have returned with cholecystitis, appendicitis, diverticulitis, and perforated ulcers. When you find yourself making the diagnosis of constipation in an elderly patient, make sure that you have considered other causes, done a reasonable evaluation, and made good follow-up plans.

4. Never trust tympanic or oral temperatures when the presence of a fever would make a difference.

References

1. Marco CA et al: Acad Emerg Med 5:1163, December 1998.
2. van Geloven AAW et al: Eur J Surg 166:866, November 2000.

Case 46

My Kingdom for a Drop of Water

Several days of nausea, vomiting, and abdominal pain brought a 77-year-old man to the emergency department. He had taken hardly anything by mouth on the day of admission. He had a history of diverticulosis and non–insulin-dependent diabetes and arrived with an oral temp of 100.8° F, a pulse rate of 120 beats/min, and a blood pressure of 105/59 mm Hg. He appeared acutely ill, and his oral membranes were quite dry. On examination the emergency physician discovered diminished bowel sounds and significant left lower quadrant tenderness, with guarding and rebound. The white blood cell count was 19,000/μl with a left shift of the differential, and the free-air series showed a small amount of subdiaphragmatic air and a nonspecific ileus. The emergency physician diagnosed peritonitis secondary to a ruptured diverticulum and quickly contacted the on-call surgeon and the patient's primary care physician, even before all lab tests were back. The surgeon promptly evaluated the patient and ordered antibiotics. Approximately 3 1/2 hours after arrival at the emergency department, the patient was wheeled directly to the surgical suite.

The necessary surgery, however, was not performed for another 2 hours because the anesthesiologist believed that the patient was too poorly hydrated to begin the procedure. Not only were the patient's membranes dry, but his creatinine level was 1.9 and his blood urea nitrogen level was 54. During the 3 ½ hours in the emergency department, the patient received less than 200 ml of normal saline. The anesthesiologist infused several liters of lactated Ringer's solution before the operation and three more during surgery. The surgeon drained an abscess and performed a sigmoid resection, and the patient did well ultimately. But the anesthesiologist called the ED director to cast aspersions upon the emergency physician for being stingy with fluids.

Analysis

The patient clearly needed hydration, which should have been started as quickly as possible. The patient came close to disaster in terms of volume depletion, and the anesthesiologist was correct to be upset. The emergency department chart contained no orders written personally by the emergency physician. They were all verbal orders, not countersigned by the physician. There were orders for lab tests, x-ray, EKG, and "IV NS," but no rate or amount had been specified. The emergency physician later recalled having asked the nurse to give the patient "a liter right away." Nothing to this effect made its way to the chart, however. The emergency physician also stated that he assumed that the surgeon, who saw the patient personally about an hour after his arrival, had dealt with the fluid issue. Although a reasonable assumption, especially since the surgeon even ordered intravenous antibiotics, it was not justified. No assumption made by the emergency physician removed him from being on the hook throughout the patient's stay.

Teaching Points

1. The only safe assumption to make about important orders for a patient in the ED is *no assumption*.

2. The best course for the emergency physician in dealing with a patient who needs intravenous fluid administration is to make an initial order that contains all of the necessary parameters: fluid type, rate of flow, and total amount.

3. Patients with peritonitis who require surgery often are dehydrated. The emergency physician is ideally placed to address hydration status carefully and expeditiously. It is part of the turf.

Case 47
Whoops

A 63-year-old woman came to the emergency department after several days of feeling weak and "dizzy." She was generally healthy, took no medications, and denied any unhealthy habits. On review of symptoms she admitted to having some headache and feeling intermittently feverish and nauseated, and she had completely lost her appetite. She denied vomiting, diarrhea, or urinary symptoms. The emergency physician did not document an adequate description of the patient's dizziness.

The patient had a low-grade temperature of 100.9° F. Her blood pressure was 138/58 mm Hg, and her pulse was 116 beats/min. The emergency physician noted an otherwise unremarkable exam. He ordered lab tests, including comprehensive chemistries. The white blood cell count was 6,800/μl without a shift, and the hemoglobin was 12.3 gm/dl. The initial chemistries were normal except for a mildly elevated blood urea nitrogen at 25 mg/dl, with normal creatinine. There was some delay in the remainder of the tests. In the meantime, the patient tolerated oral fluids well and held down the dose of meclizine that the physician ordered.

After another hour, the remainder of the lab tests were still not available, but the patient was feeling generally improved. The emergency physician discharged her with a prescription for meclizine and a diagnosis of "viral syndrome with labyrinthitis." The patient departed in the company of her husband.

A short while after she had left, the full chemistry results made their way into the emergency physician's hands. To his surprise, liver enzymes were diffusely elevated and the total bilirubin was 4.1 mg/dl. Attempts were made to call the patient back, but to no avail. Not long after returning home, she had fainted and was taken by her husband to a different emergency department, where she was admitted with a diagnosis of hepatitis and dehydration. The husband called the first hospital to complain of the misdiagnosis and how they had been "rushed in and rushed out."

Analysis

The emergency physician recalled vividly two points about this case. One was the shock of discovering significant lab abnormalities after a patient was sent home. The other was how sick he himself felt that day: "I was coming down with the flu and probably should not have even come to work that day, but we were short staffed." He added that he was probably feeling worse than most of the patients when he treated during that shift; "Ordinarily I'd never let a patient go with labs outstanding. I knew she was a little dry but she looked fine to me and was taking PO okay."

Why did he order full chemistries in the first place? "I don't know. Maybe on some subliminal level I noticed a little icterus, but it never really registered consciously." What about the diagnosis of labyrinthitis? No documentation on the chart supported the diagnosis, and no attempt was made to characterize the dizziness. "I always ask the same questions about dizziness, but for some reason I didn't write it down on her chart. Maybe I confused her with another patient. I must admit: a lot of that day is pretty hazy in my memory. I do remember getting some pressure from the nurses to free the room up. It was one of those days."

Teaching Points

1. Do not assume peripheral vertigo unless you also confirm it with *documented* clinical signs and symptoms.

2. If a lab test was ordered, make sure that you see the result before the patient leaves. Cross-check the order sheet with the results as part of the discharge routine.

3. In a patient who is clinically dehydrated, especially an older person, intravenous hydration is a safer course if discharge is planned. It gives the patient extra reserve in case he or she vomits again once or twice.

Case 48
No Entiendo

An obese 55-year-old Hispanic woman came to the emergency department one afternoon by ambulance. The triage nurse recorded the following information: "Patient complains of belly pain, constipation, and ? weak right leg. Language barrier. Pt's son translates, but minimal English."

Further information was gathered. The patient was generally healthy except for arthritis. She was currently taking acetaminophen with codeine for arthritis pain. She reported having had no bowel movement for about 4 days. She was also taking ibuprofen for pain and recently had been prescribed zolpidem for insomnia. The nursing note (but not the physician's note) also reported that the patient had a distant history of ulcers. No further mention was made of the leg weakness. The patient was afebrile, her pulse rate was 98 beats/min, her respiratory rate was 24 breaths/min, and her blood pressure 104/60 mm Hg.

The emergency physician wrote: "exam was difficult due to language barrier and obesity." Her chest was clear to auscultation, and her cardiovascular exam was normal. Her abdomen was "very obese, with normal bowel sounds, and nonspecific tenderness in lower quadrants more than upper." There was no apparent rebound tenderness or guarding, and her stool was negative for occult blood.

The emergency physician ordered routine lab tests and a kidney-ureter-bladder (KUB) x-ray. Because of the patient's obesity, the KUB required two films. They appeared to show only a great deal of stool in the colon. There were, however, some lab abnormalities. The potassium level was 3.1 mEq/L, and the bicarbonate level was 16 mEq/L. The white blood cell count was normal at 6500/μl, but there was a pronounced left shift, with 65% segmented cells and 18% band forms.

The emergency physician asked the nurses to see how she tolerated oral fluids, to administer a bottle of magnesium citrate, and to give a soap-suds enema. These instructions were followed. Because nurses said that the abdominal pain was worsening, the physician ordered an injection of ketorolac, 60 mg. Half an hour after the enema was given, the patient had a large bowel movement in the bedside commode.

The physician was informed and asked the nurse to prepare the patient for discharge. The nurse reported that the patient's son refused to take her home. The physician instructed the nurse to tell him that there were no other options. The nurse reported that the son felt that his mother was too sick to go home.

The physician was quite busy at the time. It was 20 minutes before he could reassess the situation. He found the son standing anxiously by the bedside. The patient was poorly responsive. The physician felt for her pulse. It was rapid and barely palpable. He called a code.

The patient's blood pressure was now less than 50 mm Hg by palpation. The emergency physician intubated the patient, placed a central line, and began fluids and dopamine. A postintubation chest x-ray revealed a large amount of subdiaphragmatic free air. The emergency physician consulted with a surgeon and the intensivist and transferred the patient from the emergency department to the ICU, where she died the following day.

Postmortem examination revealed frank pus in the peritoneal cavity and an apparent perforation of the duodenum, along with signs of mechanical small bowel obstruction.

An English-speaking friend of the family contacted hospital administration to raise concerns about how a patient so close to death was almost shoved onto the street.

Analysis

One of the greatest challenges of practicing emergency medicine—and the same is true for any field of medicine—lies in obtaining the necessary historical information in the face of barriers to communication and of discovering pertinent physical signs when factors such as obesity or neuropathy limit the reliability of hands-on examination. This patient had two strikes against her—a language barrier and obesity. Given such a situation, the emergency physician has no choice but to proceed with great caution, expecting the worst and looking for small clues.

Aside from the fact that a good translator should have been engaged early in this case, two not-so-small clues suggested that the patient's problem was more than simple constipation. A bicarbonate level of

16 mEq/L clearly points toward metabolic acidosis, and a bandemia of 18% suggests the presence of a major physiologic stressor. The two together raise the specter of sepsis. The emergency physician allowed his initial impression of codeine-induced constipation to minimize the importance of these red flags—so much so that he did not even mention them in his note, let alone try to explain why he chose to ignore them. Unable to delve deeply into the history because of the language barrier, he took the triage note at face value. It was a path of least resistance that led straight to an abyss.

Teaching Points

1. Abdominal pain in patients who are difficult to assess, especially the elderly and the obese, demand a more thorough evaluation and high levels of suspicion on the part of emergency physicians. Something bad is more likely to be going on and will be harder to discover.

2. Never dismiss little clues lightly, especially those suggesting the presence of metabolic acidosis.

3. Constipation in older patients, like conversion symptom or anxiety disorder, is a diagnosis of *exclusion*, to be made only after the bad actors have been duly considered.

4. Regarding language barriers: the more worrisome the complaint (e.g., abdominal pain in a obese elderly patient), the more you need a good translator.

Case 49
Sticks and Stones

A 20-year-old college student was riding his bicycle on a little-used section of a canal trail when two people suddenly pushed him to the ground and fled with his bicycle. The fall carried him into a tangle of dead bushes and resulted in several lacerations to the face. He was transported by police to the emergency department, where three lacerations to his left cheek, ranging in length from 1 to 2.5 cm, were sutured. The patient was discharged with routine follow-up instructions.

Two days later the student returned to the emergency department because the repaired wounds had begun to swell and turn red, and he had developed a low-grade fever. A different emergency physician was on duty. The patient had remarkable swelling and erythema around two of the three wounds. The physician anesthetized the area and began to remove the sutures. A fair amount of purosanguineous material immediately drained, and the physician noted that the drainage appeared to contain bits of wood or bark. He began probing the wounds and over the next several minutes removed four or five twigs and twig fragments, the largest of which measured nearly 1.8 cm in length and 3 mm in diameter. He irrigated the wounds with saline, left them open, and arranged for the patient to be admitted for intravenous antibiotic treatment.

Five days later the wounds were secondarily closed by a plastic surgeon. The eventual cosmetic result was less than desirable, and the patient contacted an attorney to pursue a lawsuit.

Analysis

The first emergency physician recalled doing a visual examination of the wounds before closing them and thought that he also recalled probing. Probing, however, was not reflected in the chart. Retained foreign bodies create a high risk for wound infections. Emergency physicians must make "exploration" an absolute and routine part of their approach to every laceration and must document the procedure. Wound exploration can be done with a finger or an instrument, but it must go beyond a casual inspection. Exploration not only discovers many foreign bodies but also establishes the depth of the wound and its proximity to other structures, such as bone, tendons, or neurovascular structures. Exploration alone does not pick up every foreign body. The clinician must exercise his or her judgment as to whether imaging studies are also warranted. Many emergency physicians, for example, x-ray every wound created by glass in the hope of picking up retained fragments. Other emergency physicians consider this approach excessive and wasteful and use a case-by-case decision-making process. Ultrasound and CT scanning also have been used to search for suspected foreign bodies. But the foreign bodies in this case should have been quite easy to discover with simple probing.

With regard to the charting of minor surgical procedures, an emergency physician's documentation should be no less thorough than that of a general surgeon for a similar case. After this incident, all physicians in the department were encouraged to chart the following for each and every laceration: (1) how the wound was prepared; (2) how the wound was anesthetized; (3) the results of exploration; (4) irrigation of the wound; and (5) with what type of suture material and with how many sutures it was closed. Good charting also leads to more accurate billing and appropriate reimbursement.

The hospital risk-management committee also raised the issue of prophylactic antibiotics when the case was reviewed. Given the nature of the wounds—tears and punctures created by wood—should the patient have been given antibiotics after the first visit? Obviously, antibiotics are of limited value when large organic foreign bodies are retained in a wound. The first step in preventing infection is to clear the wound of foreign bodies. But the general value of prophylactic antibiotics after wound closure is still debated. Recent studies failed to show a reduction in wound infection rates when antibiotics are administered prospectively.[1,2] Nonetheless, many emergency physicians administer antibiotics prophylactically for deep, contaminated wounds, especially when cosmesis is a concern. The only situation in which almost everyone agrees that preventative antibiotics are indicated is in the case of wounds created by animal or human teeth.[3,4]

The primary point remains, however, that exploration for and removal of foreign bodies are essential parts of wound care.

Teaching Points

1. All wounds require exploration.

2. Exploration and cleaning are of greater initial importance than the decision to use prophylactic antibiotics.

3. Good wound care must be documented.

References

1. Cummings P, et al: Antibiotics to prevent infection of simple wounds: A meta-analysis of randomized studies. Am J Emerg Med 13:396, 1995.
2. Stamou SC, et al: Wound infections after minor limb lacerations: Risk factors and the role of antimicrobial agents. J Trauma 46:1078, 1999.
3. Chen E, et al: Primary closure of mammalian bites. Acad Emerg Med 7:157, 2000.
4. Dankor P, et al: A study of primary closure of human bite injuries to the face. J Oral Maxillofac Surg 55:479, 1997.

Case 50
Monkeying Around

A 7-year-old girl fell on the monkey bars at school and landed astride one of the steel pipes. Her mother brought the child directly to the emergency department. The child was crying and complaining of pain. She a held partially blood soaked towel between her upper thighs and resisted lying down on the exam stretcher. Even with the help of her mother and two nurses, the male emergency physician had difficulty in examining the girl. He described seeing a laceration to the labia minora that did not appear to be bleeding at the moment, but he could not characterize the injury in more detail because of the patient's struggling. When the mother also became upset, the emergency physician ceased further efforts.

He told the patient's mother that as far as he could tell, the wound was minor. He wanted to see that the girl could urinate before she left. About half an hour later, the child urinated without obvious difficulty. A small amount of blood had dripped into the commode water, but the patient was walking without problems. The emergency physician discharged her to follow-up with her pediatrician as needed. He later stated that the mother appeared upset, but he ascribed her reaction to the general situation.

The patient continued to ooze blood from her perineum through the night. Her pediatrician referred her to a gynecologist, who also found the patient extremely uncooperative. He took her to the operating room, examined the area under conscious sedation, and placed eight sutures in the introitus region to control bleeding and close the laceration.

The mother wrote a letter to the hospital administration to complain that the emergency physician did not perform an adequate examination. Meanwhile, the gynecologist called the emergency department to warn the director that a complaint was coming and asked why the emergency physician did not sedate the child in order to examine her. It would have saved the system and the patient a lot of trouble.

Analysis

Most emergency physicians are comfortable with the practice of sedating children with either short-acting benzodiazepines, given orally or rectally, or intramuscular or intravenous ketamine for the purpose of wound repair.[1,2,3] In this situation, sedation for the purpose of examination—and then wound repair, if needed—would have been appropriate. Emergency physicians should become comfortable with one or two medications for this purpose, tailoring what they use to the policies and protocols of their institution. Emergency physicians must be aware of the potential complications of sedating medications, and appropriate resuscitation equipment must be on hand. As of the writing of this book, intramuscular ketamine appears to be the agent of choice for light sedation and axiolysis in children. It has a good safety profile, and good efficacy can minimize pain through its anesthetic effects.

Teaching Points

1. Emergency physicians who are not yet conversant with and comfortable using medications that provide anxiolysis and sedation to facilitate painful or anxiety-provoking procedures, should become so.

2. Sedation for the purpose of examination alone is appropriate; to do this is wiser than to discharge a patient who has been only partially evaluated.

3. All ED's should have protocols in place to allow the safe use of medications for this purpose.

References

1. Krauss B, et al: Sedation and analgesia for procedures in children. N Engl J Med 342:938, 2000.
2. McGlone RC, et al: An alternative to "brutacaine": A comparison of low dose intramuscular ketamine with intranasal midazolam in children before suturing. J Accid Emerg Med 15:231, 1998.
3. Green SM, et al: Intramuscular ketamine for pediatric sedation in the emergency department: Safety profile in 1,022 cases. Ann Emerg Med 31:688, June 1998.

Case 51
Super Vision

A 3-year-old boy presented to the emergency department with a
1–1.5 cm laceration on the nasal ridge directly between his eyes (the
glabella). The wound was clean and had smooth edges, but it was
deep enough to warrant closure. It seemed like a good case for the
skin adhesive recently acquired by the emergency department. While
the emergency physician was applying the skin adhesive, a drop inadvertently ran from the wound directly into the child's left eye. The
child began to cry and struggle, and the physician was unable to
obtain good closure with the glue. He injected some lidocaine and
placed four sutures.

The child's lashes, meanwhile, became glued together medially. They
were separated with some difficulty by the emergency physician with
a pair of forceps. The eye looked only slightly irritated.

The next day the parents took the child to the pediatrician because
the eye had become angry-looking. He was referred to an ophthalmologist, who diagnosed chemical conjunctivitis and made negative
comments about the care rendered by the emergency physician,
which inspired the father to write a letter of complaint. The child did
well and had no permanent damage to the eye.

Analysis

Cyanoacrylate skin adhesive has a major role in laceration repair but,
like everything else, it also has the potential for complications. Once
the child had glue in his eyes, the emergency physician may have
made the parents feel better by contacting the ophthalmologist
himself. He would have learned that any chemical irritation caused by
the adhesive should have a benign and self-limited course. He could
have transmitted this reassurance to the parents, along with routine
precautions and instructions for local care (e.g., a warm compress that
evening) that may have prevented the embarrassing and unnecessary
cascade of repeat visits and consultation.

Teaching Points

1. If you are going to use skin adhesive near the eyes, an assistant should carefully cover them with gauze pads and be prepared to sop up any adhesive that may run from the wound toward any delicate structure.

2. When an iatrogenic problem arises in the emergency department, the emergency physician should do all in his or her power to anticipate complications and concerns on the part of the patient and to initiate consultations, if needed. This approach displays an appropriate degree of concern, and smoothes the way for the patient.

Case 52
A Stitch in Time

A 3-year-old boy tripped and struck his head on a television set. He did not lose consciousness. His mother brought him to the emergency department for treatment of a small but actively bleeding parietal scalp laceration. The emergency physician examined the boy and discovered no other injuries. The laceration was quite small—only 1.5 cm—but was gaping and oozing blood. A repair was clearly in order. Rather than subject the patient to the pain of local anesthetic injections and the time required to set up a suture tray and place stitches, the physician elected instead to close it in a matter of seconds with the disposable stapling kits that the department had just received. As two nurses held the patient, he cleaned the wound with peroxide and placed two staples. The boy and his mother left the emergency department within 15 minutes of registering, and everyone seemed satisfied—except the patient, of course.

Five days later, however, when the boy arrived in the office of his pediatrician to have the staples removed, a problem arose. The pediatrician had neither the experience nor the proper equipment for removing staples. He sent his nurse to the emergency department to obtain a staple remover and instructions. When the pediatrician tried to use the staple remover, it did not seem to work properly. The child screamed and squirmed, and soon the cut was bleeding again. The pediatrician called a surgeon friend who agreed to see the child that afternoon. When the surgeon tried to remove the staples, he also encountered a great deal of screaming and squirming and discovered that the two staples seemed to have become intertwined subcutaneously. The child by now was beyond control. With the child under conscious sedation, the surgeon opened the laceration and extracted the staples, then closed the now larger wound secondarily.

The mother called the hospital medical director and explained in some detail why she did not intend to pay the bill.

Analysis

Staples are an excellent method of rapidly approximating the edges of wounds in which cosmetics are not a concern. Because they are far faster to apply than sutures, staples come into their own when the physician is treating large lacerations. For example, a 3-inch laceration to the leg or scalp, which might take 15 minutes or more to close with standard sutures, can be fixed in one or two minutes.

Smaller wounds, however, may require only a few sutures, and the ratio of time saved by using staples grows steadily smaller. In fact, for the laceration suffered by the 3-year-old boy, even if we factor in the time needed to prepare and clean the wound, the time saved by using staples is negligible.

The argument that you can actually spare the patient pain by stapling or suturing a small wound without anesthetic is also questionable. The fact is that by using buffered lidocaine and a 30-gauge needle, it is possible to numb many wounds with little discomfort to the patient—and sometimes no pain at all if one is careful and injects slowly. The advantages of working on an anesthetized wound are many. The wound can be explored and cleaned more effectively, and all lacerations, no matter how superficial, deserve at least a brief exploration along with adequate cleaning. The physician admitted that because the wound appeared minor, he did not explore and only cleaned with a dab of peroxide before applying the staple gun.

Because emergency physicians usually do not have the luxury of following up their laceration repairs, they sometimes lack a vivid understanding of the difficulties faced by those who will remove the sutures or any idea of how difficult in can be to remove sutures from small children in general. A simple step such as placing the sutures far enough from the wound edge to allow easy identification and pick-up can be a great convenience to both patient and follow-up practitioner.

As a rule, staples are not difficult to remove when placed an appropriate distance apart. If the emergency physician believes that staples are appropriate for a particular repair and knows that an outside practitioner will remove them, it is wise to give the patient a staple remover for the follow-up physician.

In the case described above, it is hard to see the justification for using staples when rapidly dissolving suture material (e.g., Vicryl Rapide) is available. Dissolving sutures are excellent for external wound closure and have the benefit of not subjecting children to another white coat.

Although it would have cost the physician five or ten extra minutes to anesthetize the wound and place dissolving sutures, this would have been the better choice.

Teaching Points

1. Avoid staples for small lacerations, especially in uncooperative patients, in whom errors of placement may occur.

2. Consider the use of rapidly dissolving sutures or cyanoacrylate glue in a patient for whom suture removal may prove cumbersome.

3. Consider the use of sedation for children before painful procedures.

4. Always keep in mind when closing wounds that someone downstream is going to have to remove the staples or sutures.

Chapter 11

Orthopedics

Case 53
Heel Thyself

A 32-year-old man riding a motorcycle swerved to avoid a car and lost control of the cycle. He was wearing a helmet and suffered no loss of consciousness and had no neck pain. After transport to the hospital in full spinal immobilization, his only complaint was bilateral ankle pain. The emergency physician examined him and ordered precautionary cervical spine films as well as views of the right and left ankles.

It was about 4 PM on Friday, but radiologists had not yet left for the weekend. The x-ray technician brought the radiologist's report, which stated that the films were negative. The emergency physician transmitted the good news to the patient, placed Ace wraps around both ankles, and prepared to discharge him with the diagnosis of bilateral ankle sprains. It was quickly discovered, however, that the patient could not bear weight, especially on the left foot. He had to be transported to his wife's car in a wheelchair. The emergency physician wrote instructions for him to follow up with his primary doctor on Monday if the pain continued and to rest and elevate his feet in the meantime.

The pain was still present on Monday, and the right foot near the heel had become grossly swollen and ecchymotic. The patient went to his family doctor who retrieved the x-rays from the hospital. The family doctor studied them and thought something looked "funny." Calcaneal views confirmed a fracture. The patient called the hospital president to complain about how the emergency doctor x-rayed his neck—which did not hurt at all—and missed the real injury. He vowed to sue if the hospital billed him and stated that they would be lucky to see his cat or dog at the same facility. The man did not return to work for over 3 months.

Analysis

Radiologists miss findings on x-rays with a fortunately low frequency. One of the reasons is their lack of contact with the patient. It is unfair to fault the emergency physician for failing to see something on x-ray that the radiologist missed, but the clinical features of a calcaneal fracture are different from those of an ankle sprain in terms of the localization of tenderness and edema. The presence of severe pain on weight-bearing, in combination with the exam, should have raised the emergency physician's suspicion. The situation did not fit the diagnosis of an ankle sprain. The severe pain on weight-bearing should have triggered a rethinking of the situation—especially in light of the mechanism of injury. Unlike a simple twist of the ankle while coming down a step, great forces can be involved in motorcycle accidents.

Teaching Points

1. Calcaneal fractures can present subtle findings on x-rays.

2. Always match the expected clinical picture against the actual clinical findings.

3. The average ankle sprain can tolerate a fair amount of weight-bearing when movement is not involved. If severe pain accompanies weight-bearing, reevaluate the situation.

Case 54
Thumbing

A 20-year-old man suffered a jamming injury to his right thumb during a football game and because of persistent pain and swelling came to the emergency department after work the following day. The emergency physician ordered an x-ray, which was negative, and placed the thumb in an alumifoam splint. The discharge instructions recommended that the splint be left in place for 3 days and that the patient follow-up with his family doctor for any problems.

The swelling and discomfort continued, and the patient saw his primary doctor about 5 days after removing the splint. The primary doctor referred the patient to an orthopedist who diagnosed "game-keeper's thumb"—a ruptured ulnar collateral ligament (UCL). He told the patient that the injury should have been suspected in the emergency department, that the thumb should have been splinted much more carefully, and that a referral should have been made sooner. The patient spent 3 weeks in a splint and afterwards underwent extensive physical therapy. Papers filed by the patient's attorney alleged that the patient—a cabinetmaker by trade—was left with residual functional impairment of the thumb.

The emergency physician's liability carrier believed that the patient's chart was too incompletely documented to allow a reasonable defense of the case, and a settlement was made.

Analysis

Like occult carpal scaphoid/navicular fractures and occult fractures of the radial head, traumatic rupture of the UCL of the interphalangeal joint of the thumb can easily be missed and carries the potential for long-term disability. When dealing with thumb injuries, the emergency physician must check for tenderness over the ulnar collateral ligament and assess the stability of the joint. If there is any question of an injury to the ligament, the thumb should be carefully immobilized, the patient instructed about possible complications, and a good follow-up plan arranged. All of these steps must be documented.

As always, emergency physicians must show they took the worst-case scenario into due consideration and took adequate precautions on behalf of the patient's well-being.

Teaching Points

1. Always check for UCL injury when examining injured thumbs.

2. Always document that you did so.

3. If you have any suspicion of a gamekeeper's thumb injury, adequately splint and refer the patient for definitive follow-up.

Case 55
Come Again?

A 25-year-old woman injured her left ring finger while playing volley-ball. She came to the emergency department the next day and was triaged directly to radiology. When she returned to the emergency department, the emergency physician examined her and read the x-ray, which was negative. He diagnosed a sprain, splinted the digit, and discharged the patient with instructions to wear the splint for 3 days.

Four days later the patient visited her family doctor because the swelling and pain were no better. The family physician got the x-ray report and discovered that the x-ray technician had isolated the middle—not the ring—finger for evaluation. An x-ray that focused on the proper digit showed an avulsion fracture that was visible only laterally.

The patient filed a formal complaint with the hospital and challenged her bill as well as the emergency physician's competence.

Analysis

The successful practice of emergency medicine is a highly interde-pendent art. Every day we make small and large decisions based on assumptions that other departments and our many colleagues have done their job correctly. Such assumptions are necessary. We cannot—and should not need to—redo the work of others. On the other hand, it takes essentially no time or energy to validate certain assumptions. We should make it a habit when reading radiographs to make sure that name on the study matches the patient under consid-eration and that the correct side and proper body part received the proper attention.

The emergency physician's physical description of the injury on the chart—"marked swelling with ecchymosis"—also suggested that something more than a sprain may have been present. Even if an x-ray of the proper finger had been negative, the patient would have had at least a significant ligamentous injury. More definite follow-up parameters should have been given.

Teaching Points

1. Always assume that the wrong patient's x-ray is in the folder and that the technician x-rayed the wrong area. In other words, demonstrate trust in your colleagues, from consultants to technicians, but remember that they are only human.

2. If, despite normal x-rays, the clinical appearance of an injury appears more significant than a simple sprain or contusion and may bear greater risk of complication, instruct the patient to obtain definite follow-up.

3. This approach is not "practicing medicine with a lawyer on your shoulder." It is simply giving good care.

Case 56
From a Different Angle

A healthy 28-year-old man slipped on his daughter's toy and fell down a flight of stairs. He came to the emergency department the next morning complaining only of severe low back pain, with no radiation into the legs and no leg weakness or numbness. On examination, the emergency physician discovered tenderness in the mid-lumbar region. Concerned about the possibility of a compression fracture, he gave the patient a shot of meperidine and sent him to radiology for lumbar spine films.

Because it was Saturday morning, no radiologist was on duty. The emergency physician had recently attended an M&M conference in which a missed L1 compression fracture was presented, so he scanned the lumbar spine films with special attention to the thoracolumbar junction. He saw no sign of compression fractures and read the films as negative. He discharged the patient with an analgesic prescription and recommendations for several days of bed rest.

The x-ray received a formal reading by the radiologist on Monday, at which time transverse process fractures of L2 and L3 were discovered. A different emergency physician on duty called the patient, told him about the misreading, and asked him to return. The man, however, had already seen his primary physician because of worsening pain, which had lateralized to some extent in the left flank region. A urinalysis showed microscopic hematuria. The primary physician admitted the patient for pain control, orthopedic consultation, and an abdominal CT to check for renal damage. The CT was negative, and the man had an uncomplicated two-day hospitalization.

The man's family, however, called the emergency department to complain and subsequently refused to pay the emergency department bill.

Analysis

Transverse process fractures of the lumbar spine are relatively uncommon injuries, usually caused by a direct force, (e.g., a fall onto the edge of a stair). Fortunately, isolated lumbar transverse process fractures are usually stable and are not associated with neurologic or visceral organ injuries. They indicate, however, that a significant degree of force was involved and therefore mandate a thorough evaluation of the abdomen and distal neurologic status.

Transverse process fractures are also relatively easy to see on plain films, if the examiner is looking for them. The problem is that emergency physicians see hundreds of lumbar spine films before they encounter a transverse process fracture. Looking for them must become habitual.

If the emergency physician had detected the transverse process fracture, he might easily have spared the patient an unnecessary admission and probably an unnecessary CT scan. Given the forces necessary to create a lumbar transverse process fracture, it is arguably always reasonable to check for hematuria. If the emergency physician finds hematuria, the next step remains a matter of clinical judgment. Renal contusions are common and usually benign. Which patients deserve evaluation for a more serious kidney injury, such as pedicle avulsion, depends up various considerations, including the amount of force involved, associated injuries, and degree of abdominal discomfort. Always keep in mind that the most devastating renal injuries may not display hematuria, gross or otherwise.

A patient with a transverse process fracture, microscopic hematuria, and a completely normal abdominal exam probably does not need further imaging to assess for possible kidney damage. Follow-up of the renal situation, of course, is necessary. When follow-up can be arranged prospectively, as opposed to after-the-fact in the setting of a missed injury, excessive responses by downstream physicians as well as an excess of embarrassment for the emergency department are less likely to occur.

Teaching Points

1. You must search for transverse process fractures in all x-rays of the lumbar spine.

2. The presence of such an injury should trigger a reevaluation for possible neurologic or visceral organ injury.

Case 57
Dem Bones

A 15-year-old boy suffered a leg injury during baseball and was brought to the emergency department for evaluation. The exact mechanism of injury was uncertain, but remarkable tenderness and swelling were present over the distal tibia. Ankle x-rays demonstrated a nondisplaced medial malleolar fracture. The patient was splinted and discharged. On follow up with the orthopedist two days later, a proximal fibular fracture was also discovered.

Analysis

Unlike its more common cousin the distal fibular fracture (which is usually an isolated injury in terms of bony structures), distal tibial fractures are often associated with proximal fibular fractures. Whenever you see a medial malleolar fracture, palpate the fibula carefully and x-ray it if any tenderness is discovered.

Teaching Point

Always suspect a proximal fibular fracture when you find a medial malleolar (distal tibial) fracture.

Case 58
The Laying On of Hands

A 6-year-girl was brought to the emergency department on the day after a fall on the playground. The emergency nurse who triaged her wrote on the chart: "No obvious injuries. Complains of some wrist pain. Parents anxious—always here with minor problems."

It was a busy day for the emergency physician on duty because the midlevel provider scheduled to cover the fast track had called in sick and no replacement was available. After a wait of some 3 hours, the patient was taken to a treatment room and the emergency physician arrived shortly thereafter. According to a later statement from the parents, the doctor did not cross the threshold of the room. He asked questions from the doorway, looked at the patient from 6 feet away, and told the parents that nothing was wrong.

The next day the parents took the child to a pediatrician, who ordered an x-ray of the wrist and discovered a minor buckle fracture of the distal radius. Hearing the story of the emergency physician's behavior, the pediatrician wrote a letter of complaint to the vice president of medical affairs.

When the emergency physician was interviewed, he stated that because of the many sick patients in the department that day, he had relied on the nurse's evaluation. He said that he was angry for being "called on the carpet" for such a minor issue. If the hospital were really worried about quality of care, they would arrange reliable back-up coverage when physician extenders in the fast track "decide to play hooky."

The vice president of medical affairs responded that it would not have cost the emergency physician any extra time to have stepped into the room and examined the patient while he was talking to the parents. A brief argument ensued. The emergency physician's contract was not renewed several months later.

Analysis

The buckle fracture (also called torus fracture) is a common orthopedic injury of childhood in which a region of bony cortex crumples in response to a longitudinal force, creating a circumferential ring of disruption, usually without significant angulation. The bone most frequently involved is the distal radius, and the most common mechanism is a fall on an outstretched hand. This benign fracture often presents a day or more after the injury, when delayed swelling and persistent pain raise the parents' level of concern. Buckle fractures can present with relatively little swelling and no obvious deformity. Unless the clinician palpates in an effort to localize the tenderness, visual evaluation alone may yield no clues.

The emergency physician allowed the frustrations of a busy, short-handed day to lure him into the trap of minimizing the problem. The triage nurse's unnecessary comment about the parent's low threshold for misusing the emergency department set him up, and he took the bait. The child had an absolutely classic buckle fracture to the upper extremity: she arrived on the day after a fall with wrist pain. By any measure an exam was warranted.

It may not be a big deal to miss a minor fracture, but it means inconvenience to the patient, expenditure of additional resources, embarrassment to the hospital and emergency department, and, in rare cases, loss of someone's job.

Teaching Points

1. Buckle fractures are common in childhood and usually involve the distal radius.

2. Patients with buckle fractures often do not seek care until a day or so after the injury.

3. Buckle fractures are easy to miss unless the physician keeps a reasonable index of suspicion.

4. Missing a problem owing to "examination at a distance" does not endear the physician to patients, family, administrators, or colleagues.

Case 59
By the Collar

A collision between a two-and-a-half-year-old girl and the family dog resulted in a fall. She pointed to the right side of her chest when asked where it hurt. The emergency physician auscultated and palpated her chest. Although the chest was a little tender superiorly on the right, the findings seemed benign and nonspecific. Further examination revealed no signs of head or neck trauma. The abdomen was soft, and examination of the extremities revealed only minor discomfort on range-of-motion testing of the right shoulder. By then the child was upset, and it was hard to draw conclusions.

The emergency physician recommended acetaminophen for pain and told the parents that he could find nothing seriously wrong. The parents were not comforted, and visited the family doctor on the following day. The family doctor ordered a chest x-ray, and the radiologist discovered a fracture of the right clavicle. The parents called the emergency department to complain.

Analysis

Although they usually have a benign clinical course, missed clavicle fractures are not a benign event to parents who receive a bill for wasted time in the emergency department. The clavicle is the most commonly fractured bone in the human body. Almost any type of fall that exerts lateral pressure on the shoulder transmits force directly to this relatively slender, already bowed structure and may cause it to snap, usually in midsection. This injury is common in young children and can be difficult to diagnose from verbal clues alone in a preverbal population. A high index of suspicion is needed when there is any suggestion of pain near the collarbone. The emergency physician should attempt to palpate the clavicle itself, and if the slightest suspicion of tenderness is found, an x-ray is indicated. The physician in this case did not document palpation of the clavicle and could not remember definitely having done so.

The take-home message is clear: to avoid missing clavicle fractures, the emergency physician must keep a high index of suspicion for this common and easy-to-overlook diagnosis. It should be considered in any child who has suffered a fall. If the child is preverbal and exam findings raise even the slightest suspicion, an x-ray is indicated.

Teaching Points

1. Maintain a high index of suspicion for clavicle fractures in all children who suffer falls and have any discomfort in the shoulder or upper chest.

2. If you decide not to x-ray, make sure that the patient has a definite follow-up plan in case the symptoms do not quickly resolve.

60
Don't Worry About It

One Friday afternoon, a 59-year-old construction worker presented to the emergency department after a pile of railroad ties toppled off a forklift and pinned his legs. On arrival he had pain and bruising mainly to his left thigh. His vital signs were normal, the leg had generally good range of movement, and the distal neurovascular exam was negative. The emergency physician ordered x-rays of the pelvis, hip, and femur, all of which were read as negative. Nonetheless, weight-bearing on the left leg was quite uncomfortable, especially with movement involving the hamstring muscle.

The emergency physician gave the patient a tablet of hydrocodone with acetaminophen, a prescription for 20 more tablets, and a note to remain off work and at rest for two days. The patient was discharged with instructions to follow-up in 3 days at the occupational medicine clinic.

By 11 PM the pain in the left thigh was so severe that the patient's wife called the emergency department for advice. The nurse who answered the call put the wife on hold, retrieved the chart, and spoke briefly with the physician on duty. She told the wife that the x-rays had been read by the radiologist and were normal and that her husband needed to keep elevating the leg and taking the pain medication, doubling the dosage if necessary. If the pain did not improve in two days, she should bring him back for evaluation.

The patient returned to the emergency department approximately 36 hours later, still in severe pain despite medication. His left thigh was markedly swollen, tense, and tender, and distal pulses were difficult to identify. The emergency physician on duty empirically diagnosed a compartment syndrome and contacted the orthopedist on call. The diagnosis was confirmed by manometric testing, and the man was taken to the operating room. Substantial damage to muscle tissue required extensive debridement.

The man and his wife engaged an attorney and ultimately received a large settlement, largely on the basis of the unfortunate advice given to the patient's wife.

Analysis

Telephone calls to the emergency department for advice have long been recognized as dangerous events from a liability standpoint—especially when the call is from a patient previously seen in the department. Such calls should be viewed as opportunities to make sure that all went well with the visit. They are great opportunities to reinforce follow-up directions and to assess for unexpected problems. Staff members dealing with such calls must have a low threshold for inviting the patient back if symptoms are worsening. Policy should mandate notification of the physician on duty when a recent patient calls with progression of symptoms. The physician should review the chart and make an informed decision about whether this patient needs reevaluation.

In this case, the emergency physician on duty remembered only that the nurse asked whether a patient with a contusion and increased pain could take two pain pills at once. It may be understandable how such a benign query aroused no suspicion—but emergency physicians should be wary of phrases such as "worse pain."

The simplest way to prevent such problems is to tell every prior patient who calls the emergency department to return for reassessment. But this approach is overkill and probably would never be uniformly applied. On the other hand, the worst possible outcome when patients return is that they leave with a better understanding of the problem and some reassurance.

In this case, a complication might have been prevented by strict instructions for the patient to *return immediately* if the pain worsened.

Teaching Points

1. Be suspicious for the development of compartment syndrome in crush injuries to extremities.

2. Patients at risk for compartment syndromes should receive strict instructions to return at the first sign of worsening pain.

3. When patients call back after an initial emergency department visit with progression of symptoms, do not miss this opportunity to catch a complication before it evolves beyond repair.

Case 61
The Tail of the Horse

A 41-year-old man visited his family doctor with complaints of back pain that occasionally shot down his right leg. He was obese but otherwise in good health and had never experienced back problems in the past. He worked at an auto parts store and frequently carried boxes that weigh 30 to 40 pounds. The family physician recommended 2 days of bed rest and prescribed Voltaren and cyclobenzaprine. Ten days later, he returned to the doctor's office. Although he had experienced some improvement at first, now he could hardly get out of bed. He seemed to be moving around fairly well, however, and the family doctor sent him for plain films of the lumbosacral spine, which were negative. He then wrote the man a prescription for cyclobenzaprine and hydrocodone with acetaminophen.

That night he came to the emergency department for the first of three visits. He complained of severe pain in the lumbar area and varying pain in the right thigh. Leg strength was normal, but pinprick sensation was slightly diminished in the right lateral thigh. Deep tendon reflexes were normal. Any effort to raise the legs created low back spasms. The emergency physician documented that the patient had no complaints of bladder or bowel dysfunction. The physician performed a rectal exam, noting in the chart that sphincter tone was normal.

The patient was given an injection of meperidine for pain. After 1 hour, he felt good enough to go home for bed rest. He was discharged with a prescription for a stronger hydrocodone/acetaminophen combination, along with more cyclobenzaprine, and instructions to call his primary care provider for a follow-up appointment.

The patient visited the family doctor 2 days later. He required a cane to walk into the office, because the pain in his right thigh and buttocks was severely exacerbated by movement. After the patient turned pale and seemed about to faint in the waiting room, the family physician called 911 and had the patient taken to the emergency department by ambulance.

A second emergency physician evaluated the patient. The chart shows that he was again asked about bowel or bladder dysfunction and replied in the negative. According to the chart, he complained of some numbness in the right buttocks that moved downward toward the groin area. There were no motor or deep tendon reflex deficits. The emergency physician ordered an injection of meperidine for pain. An hour later the man felt reasonably comfortable and was discharged to bed rest at home.

By 10 PM the back, thigh, and buttock pain had worsened. Other symptoms included severe crampy, burning suprapubic pain and inability to urinate, along with a sense of numbness throughout the groin. The patient returned to the emergency department by ambulance. The nurse's triage note indicated that the chief complaint was "can't urinate."

A new emergency physician was on duty. Percussion of the abdomen revealed a distended bladder. The back pain was noted, as was a positive straight leg raising sign on the right, but the chart contained no further mention of neurologic testing. A rectal exam was not performed. The emergency physician ordered the patient to be "straight-cathed," and 700 ml of clear urine was drained. The physician also ordered an injection of meperidine and discharged the patient to follow-up on the next day with his family doctor. The discharge diagnosis was "Urinary Retention Secondary to Cyclobenzaprine." The family physician arranged for the patient to have an MRI, which demonstrated a large central disc herniation at the L5–S1 level. The patient was admitted to the neurosurgical center with a diagnosis of cauda equina syndrome. He was taken within several hours of admission to the operating room where a huge segment of extruded disc was removed and the neural canal decompressed.

The patient, however, was left with a urogenic bladder and sexual dysfunction. The hospital administration learned of the case from the man's attorney.

Analysis

Of the handful of truly serious pitfalls that an emergency physician faces, a missed cauda equina syndrome—like a missed premonitory (herald) subarachnoid bleed—is among the most serious. Early recognition can avert a disastrous outcome for the patient. By focusing on urinary retention instead of its potentially direct relationship with the back pain, the third emergency physician missed a rare opportunity. Urinary retention secondary to the anticholinergic effects of cyclobenzaprine was certainly in the differential diagnosis, but the emergency physician closed the door too quickly. He did not consider the worst-case scenario. A patient with back pain and autonomic dysfunction has cauda equina compression until proved otherwise. If this fairly uncommon condition is not considered, it will be missed. Emergency physicians can go years without seeing a case, but every patient with back pain must be asked about the presence of "saddle" anesthesia and bowel or bladder dysfunction (usually fecal incontinence and urinary retention). A rectal exam and perineal sensory testing should be done if there is any concern.

In general, it is difficult to study this case without asking why it took so long for the patient to receive imaging and a referral. The patient's second visit to the family physician, during which he nearly fainted from the pain, should probably have been the point at which consultation was obtained. The family practitioner, however, elected merely to send the patient to the emergency department. It is a common situation—primary care providers triage a patient to the emergency department for reasons of logistics. Although this practice certainly does not constitute abandonment of the patient by the family doctor, it often means that the emergency physician becomes by default the provider responsible for making important decisions about further consultations and referrals. The second emergency physician discharged the patient, bouncing him back to the family doctor, even though the numbness in the buttocks and groin area justified, at a minimum, contact with a spine specialist or arranging contact with the specialist through the family doctor. This course of action almost certainly would have led to an imaging study being performed earlier.

The third physician unquestionably dropped the ball, but the second one should have been more aggressive.

Teaching Points

1. Cauda equina syndrome can be easily missed if the physician does not ask about bowel or bladder dysfunction and perineal sensory changes.

2. Always perform a rectal exam to check sphincter tone if cauda equina compression is suspected.

3. If you have reason to believe that the primary care provider is not sufficiently aggressive in the evaluation of a clinical problem, you may consider obtaining independent consultation. The most that the primary care provider can do is to complain. Usually he or she is thankful that you took the initiative.

Case 62
Meddling with the Occult

A retarded 43-year-old man living in a group home was found sitting on the floor next to his bed. He said that he had fallen out of bed and that his left hip hurt too much to stand. The supervisor helped him to his feet; he was able to walk to the front porch but refused to go any further. An ambulance was called.

On arrival at the emergency department, the man was still complaining of pain in the left hip area, but he was able to get out of bed and use a bedside commode, according to the nurse's note. The nurse's note also mentioned that the patient had a history of attention-seeking behavior. The emergency physician examined him and noted no signs of injury other than general discomfort to palpation in the left pelvic and hip area. Bilateral hip range of motion seemed reasonably full, although the patient felt some discomfort on the left side. An x-ray of the pelvis and left hip were read as negative by the radiologist. Before discharging the man, the emergency physician personally got him off the stretcher and walked him around the room. The patient favored the left leg but seemed to get around reasonably well. He was discharged with instructions to use a walker as needed.

Five evenings later the man was brought back to the emergency department. He was still limping and complaining of pain in the left hip. His symptoms were not improving according to the group home staff member. A different emergency physician obtained the previous chart and examined the patient. The exam findings were identical. The previous films were brought to the emergency department, and the physician looked them over himself, confirming that they were perfectly normal. He prescribed acetaminophen with propoxyphene and discharged the patient to rest at home for several days. He instructed the patient to follow-up with the primary doctor and to continue using the walker as needed.

That evening the patient collapsed while walking down the hall to the bathroom and arrived in the emergency department screaming about pain in the left hip. This time the x-rays revealed an obvious fracture of the left femoral neck.

Analysis

Occult hip fracture is quite common but usually is seen in the elderly. A rule of thumb is that if the mechanism of action fits and the hip hurts, the patient has a fracture until proved otherwise. The patient should be kept from bearing weight for a week or so, and x-rays should be repeated.[1] Alternatively, a different kind of imaging can be performed. Although bone scans have been the traditional method for detecting occult hip fractures, MRI may be the more useful technique.[2,3]

During the patient's first visit, the emergency physician should have considered an MRI. This option was even more important during the second visit.

Teaching Points

1. Always suspect occult hip fracture.

2. Such patients should be considered candidates for either admission or discharge without weight-bearing. Good outpatient follow-up and subsequent imaging are mandatory.

References

1. Alba E, et al: Occult fractures of the femoral neck. Am J Emerg Med 10:64, 1992.
2. Evans PD, et al: Comparison of MRI with bone scanning for suspected hip fracture in elderly patients. J Bone Joint Surg 76B:158, 1994.
3. Pandey, R, et al: The role of MRI in the diagnosis of occult hip fractures. Injury 29:61, 1998.

Case 63
Sweating the Little Stuff

An intoxicated 41-year-old man walked into the emergency department half an hour after being involved in a roll-over accident with his pick-up truck. He had been the belted driver and sole occupant and denied any loss of consciousness or neck pain. However, he had a large laceration on his forehead, diffuse facial abrasions, pain and swelling of the left ankle, pain with inspiration in the lower left anterior chest, and tenderness in the left upper abdomen. His right index finger was obviously dislocated at the proximal interphalangeal joint.

Based on the mechanism of injury, the visible signs of head injury, and the patient's intoxication, the emergency physician elected to do an especially careful evaluation. CT of the head and abdomen were performed, as well as plain x-rays of the chest, left ankle, and right index finger. The CT scans were negative, as were the ankle and chest films, but the finger x-ray showed dislocation and a volar-plate fracture of the middle phalanx.

The emergency physician performed digital block anesthesia, reduced the finger dislocation, and applied a splint. Meanwhile, the lab tests returned. Everything was normal except an elevated blood alcohol and the presence of microscopic hematuria. (A forensic blood alcohol level also had been drawn at the request of law enforcement officers.)

The patient was observed in the emergency department through the rest of the night. He remained stable and was discharged with a family member on the next morning with instructions to follow-up with his family physician for a repeat urinalysis and evaluation of the finger injury. No postreduction film had been ordered.

The patient did not followup for approximately 3 weeks. By that time his index finger was locked in flexion. A lawsuit was filed, contending that the finger dislocation had not been properly reduced and that the follow-up instructions had been too vague. The emergency physician's liability carrier settled the case despite the physician's objections that his actions were defensible.

Analysis

It seems highly unfair that the emergency physician should bear the onus of a settled claim when he had clearly expended great and intelligent effort to rule out any life-threatening problem. However, the little things often catch us. Wise practice dictates a postreduction x-ray. It is the standard of care, even though it may seem unnecessary. A close look at the patient's chart reveals other issues and makes more understandable the insurance company's decision to avoid the risk of a trial. In addition to the lack of a postreduction film, the finger injury and treatment were poorly documented. The entire description read: "index finger reduced under digital block, splinted." The chart contained no mention of the return of range of motion after reduction, no mention of neurovascular status or joint stability, and no mention of splinting material or splinting position. The discharge instructions said only to "keep splint on and see your doctor for follow-up."

Skimpy documentation will undercut any defense that an emergency physician might make. It basically leaves the physician at the mercy of a hostile patient's recall.

Teaching Points

1. Remember to sweat the little things. The case is not complete until all aspects have been adequately addressed.

2. Postreduction films are a standard of care.

3. After joint reduction, always document the return of normal appearance and appropriate functional attributes.

4. An orthopedist's documentation of joint immobilization always contains a description of the material used and the position in which the affected part was splinted. Emergency physicians are held to the same standard.

5. Follow-up instructions for dislocations, as for any joint or bone injury with the potential for adverse sequelae, should be highly specific.

Case 64
Tail Wags Dog

A 21-year-old woman who was six-and-a-half months pregnant was the belted front-seat passenger of a car that was struck by a pick-up truck on the driver's side. The patient did not lose consciousness, but she had a small abrasion on her left forehead. She arrived in the emergency department by ambulance in full spinal immobilization, complaining of pain in the right knee and considerable crampy lower abdominal pain. The driver of the car, her husband, suffered a fractured left wrist and no other injuries.

The emergency physician examined the patient, who was also complaining about the hardness of the backboard. He found no other signs of head injury. She had full movement and sensation in the extremities, despite some pain and swelling over the left patella. The patient had no neck pain. The physician stated that he carefully removed the collar while someone held the patient's head and then palpated the cervical spine, which was completely free of tenderness. He then began gentle range-of-motion testing of the neck. The neck moved freely without generating discomfort. He then palpated the thoracic and lumbar spines; discovering no pain or tenderness, he completely removed the cervical collar and got the patient off the backboard.

Her lower abdomen was somewhat tense, but the abdomen was primarily remarkable for intermittent sharp pains. There was no vaginal bleeding or obvious fluid leakage. After an x-ray of the left knee, the physician asked an obstetric nurse to place a fetal monitoring device on the patient. He then called the patient's obstetrician, who was located about 30 miles away. The obstetrician asked the emergency physician to transfer the patient to the medical center for overnight observation if indeed she was as stable as he said. The center had a neonatal intensive care unit in the event that she delivered.

The patient agreed to this plan, the results of fetal monitoring were unremarkable, and shortly afterwards the patient left by ambulance.

Two days later, the emergency department director received a call from the new chief of surgery at the accepting medical center. The patient had been received initially by the trauma service. The trauma resident had lodged a formal complaint against the transferring hospital because the patient's cervical spine had not been cleared radiographically. By the time she arrived at the medical center, she was complaining of neck stiffness.

The chief of surgery intimated that he was considering filing a notice of COBRA violation with the Health Care Financing Administration, because "this happened all the time."

Analysis

Many trauma centers have protocols that mandate the performance of cervical spine films in any patient who presents to the emergency department with spinal immobilization placed by prehospital care providers. The rationale is simple and understandable: it reduces the likelihood that a trainee will miss any significant problem. Surgical house-staff (not so much emergency medicine residents) indoctrinated in this "wisdom" often believe that it is "impossible to clinically clear" a neck and that occult cervical spine fractures are lurking in every patient.

But reality is different. Good evidence indicates that it is perfectly reasonable to clear a neck by examination if a patient has no head injury and no neck pain or tenderness, is not intoxicated, is neurologically intact, and has no significant "distracting" injury elsewhere.[1] There is some disagreement about the exact incidence of occult cervical spine fractures, but most authors agree they are uncommon, if not rare; at best, the situation does not justify x-raying the cervical spine of every asymptomatic patient involved in any injury that conceivably could harm the neck.

The emergency physician not only cleared the patient's neck properly, he documented his actions well. A letter to that effect was sent to the chief of surgery.

Teaching Points

Clinical clearance of cervical spines according to NEXUS criteria:

- Completely alert patient
- No midline neck tenderness
- No neurologic deficits

- No intoxication
- No distracting injuries

References

1. Hofman JR, et al: Validity of a set of clinical criteria to rule out injury to the cervical spine in patients with blunt trauma. N Engl J Med 343:94, 2000.

Case 65
She's Back Again

A 56-year-old obese women fell at work while lifting some boxes onto a shelf and presented two days later to the emergency department complaining of diffuse spinal pain from neck to tailbone. The patient had a history of previous back problems, which usually resolved with rest and ibuprofen. The initial history on the chart did not describe the mechanism of injury in detail.

The patient described the pain as severe and said that it seemed to move everywhere up and down. The emergency physician's exam uncovered no obvious sensory deficits or specific area of muscle weakness. The physician noted on the chart that the patient was difficult to examine because of anxiety and diffuse symptoms. But her lumbar spine seemed the most tender. He ordered a lumbosacral spine x-ray, which was read as normal, and discharged the patient with a prescription for ibuprofen and cyclobenzaprine.

Two weeks later the patient returned to the emergency department. She reported increased back and neck pain and also described feeling weak in both arms and legs. Three days earlier her primary care physician had prescribed hydrocodone, crutches, and two more days of bed rest. She now reported that it was impossible to use the crutches, because her right arm felt too weak to support her. A different emergency physician was on duty and later reported that the patient was a "tough historian," anxious and weepy, who angered easily during the evaluation. The patient was either unable or unwilling to complete tasks during her evaluation. On review of systems, the patient reported several recent episodes of urinary incontinence and said that she was having trouble with giving herself insulin injections in the thigh because she could not feel the needle.

Repeat lumbosacral spine films were negative. The patient was given a shot of meperidine and lorazepam and told to follow up with her primary doctor. The patient was then carried by several members of the staff and placed in the back seat of her car.

The patient sought treatment at a tertiary facility several days later because she could no longer move her right arm and leg. An emergency MRI revealed a significant cervical disk herniation. Despite surgical intervention and aggressive physical therapy, the patient was left with disabling neurologic deficits.

Analysis

Certain patients are more difficult to evaluate than others. Overlying fatty tissue obscures tenderness, and high levels of anxiety make findings unreliable and frustrating to localize. The patient fit into both categories. In retrospect, the second emergency department visit was associated with definite clues that the problem was more serious than a back strain—the upper extremity weakness, urinary incontinence, and hypesthesia in the thigh. The emergency physician who evaluated the patient during the second visit ordinarily performed her work in a thorough and competent manner. Clearly, the signs pointing to a more serious problem were obscured to some extent by the patient's anxiety.

Nonetheless, the combination of both upper and lower extremity complaints, along with incontinence, should have triggered thoughts of an ominous process in the neck.

The lack of a description in both emergency department records of the initial mechanism is also problematic. Providers at the tertiary care center learned that the patient had fallen off a step-ladder and had hyperflexed her neck when the back of her head struck a stack of boxes. This information might have heightened the suspicions of both emergency physicians for a problem above the back.

This case reinforces the point that return visits to the emergency department represent a great opportunity to find pathology either overlooked or not present to an appreciable degree on the first visit. Such patients deserve careful attention.

The second emergency physician should not have discharged a patient with such difficulty in ambulation. The physician stated later that she felt certain that the patient was malingering. This assumption is rarely safe in the emergency department. Malingering must be a diagnosis of exclusion.

In any case, that picture of the patient being "dumped in a car" did not play well before the jury.

Teaching Points

1. A good history of the mechanism of injury is the first step in avoiding missteps.

2. Be especially vigilant with the patient who returns with worsening symptoms.

3. Be especially vigilant with patients who are difficult to evaluate because of obesity and a high background level of anxiety or anger.

4. Bowel or bladder dysfunction in combination with spinal pain indicates nerve compression until proved otherwise.

Case 66
Back to the Future

A healthy 52-year-old woman arrived at the emergency department in full spinal immobilization after her car was rear-ended at low speed by another vehicle. She had not been wearing a seat belt and had a small bump on her forehead. She also complained of pain in the right knee but had been ambulatory at the scene. She denied loss of consciousness. She had no headache, nausea, or dizziness. She denied neck discomfort and described the pain in her knee as mild.

It was a busy day, and all of the rooms were full. The patient was lifted onto a stretcher in the hallway where the emergency physician evaluated her shortly afterward. He ordered x-rays of the cervical spine and knee. The patient spent the next hour and a half immobilized on the backboard, waiting her turn for radiology. At some point during this interlude, she began to develop low back pain. When the technician finally came to wheel her to the radiology suite, the back discomfort was so pronounced that she told the technician, who called the emergency physician and received orders to add views of the lumbosacral spine.

The x-rays were negative, and the emergency physician discharged the patient with instructions to rest for two days and take ibuprofen for pain.

The patient was dissatisfied with her care and called the hospital administrator to complain. She felt that she did not need x-rays and that lying on the board caused her back to hurt for several days. She said that if she developed cancer from the x-rays, she would know whom to sue.

The same physician was involved on the same busy day with another complaint, which was picked up on a routine patient survey:

> We waited three hours while my son was restrained on a board and taped to sandbags. It was a truly nightmarish experience. The ED doctor and staff were more concerned about discussing where their next dinner came from. I had to scream at them for attention. There could not be a more inhospitable place than your ER.

The times were checked against the chart. The patient was on the board for a little under two hours, but the exact time hardly seems to negate the issue. His x-rays were also negative.

Analysis

The need for prehospital care personnel to immobilize patients with potential spinal injury is unquestionable. But once the patient arrives in the emergency department, several other issues are also unquestionable:

1. Most patients who arrive on backboards do not have spinal injuries.

2. Nearly all patients left on the backboard for a long enough period will develop spinal pain, especially in the low back.

3. A person in full spinal immobilization who vomits and is unattended may be in serious trouble.

Emergency physicians should be adept at safely "clearing" cervical spines using the NEXUS criteria (as described in the "Tail Wags Dog" case above). Furthermore, every effort should be made to clear the spine, either clinically or by x-ray, as quickly as possible. Healthy subjects uniformly develop back pain after spending between half an hour and an hour and 20 minutes on a backboard. This iatrogenic pain can lead to unnecessary imaging.[1] But worse than unnecessary discomfort is the fact that collared, taped, strapped, and back-boarded people are at risk for aspiration. These concerns—discomfort and airway risk—should compel us to clear such patients clinically or by x-ray as quickly as possible. If time does not permit a full evaluation, at least address the issue of whether continued immobilization is needed. Almost always it is not. In some emergency departments a back-boarded patient goes to the head of the list (or very close) in terms of priority. This policy is probably wise.

Teaching Points

1. Patients brought to the emergency department in spinal immobilization should not be left on the backboard any longer than absolutely necessary.

2. Patients left on backboards for prolonged periods invariably have back pain. Ask whether the pain began before or after placement on the board before deciding that the patient needs lumbosacral spinal films.

3. Patients in full immobilization are at risk for aspiration if they vomit. If the immobilization is truly necessary, make sure that the patient is directly observed, or has access to a call bell to summon assistance.

Reference

1. Lerner EB, et al: Duration of patient immobilization in the ED. Am J Emerg Med 18:28, 2000.

Case 67
ABCs

A 59-year-old man came to the emergency department with severe respiratory compromise. He was taking multiple medications for chronic obstructive pulmonary disease (COPD), including home nebulizers and oxygen. The emergency physician on duty was trained in family practice with nearly 5 years of emergency medicine experience in smaller hospitals. On arrival the patient was in extreme respiratory distress—profoundly cyanotic and not far from respiratory arrest. The emergency physician immediately attempted to perform orotracheal intubation, but the patient was conscious enough to resist vigorously. After sedating the patient with lorazepam, his attempts were still unsuccessful. The hypopharynx was now full of blood. The emergency physician ordered the respiratory technician to begin bag-mask ventilation and paged anesthesiology.

Fortunately, the anesthesiologist was just finishing up his last case of the day. He came to the emergency department and began his own intubation attempts, which did not go smoothly. When the anesthesiologist was finally able to place a tube, the patient's oxygen saturation, already below 80%, continued to worsen. Concluding that the tube was in the esophagus, the anesthesiologist extubated the patient to try again. At this point, the hospital's only intensivist, known as the "airway king," passed through the emergency department. He promptly intubated the patient, who by now was unconscious and flaccid. A chest x-ray shortly thereafter demonstrated a possible pneumomediastinum.

Based on the overall situation, including the possibility that iatrogenic esophageal perforation had caused the pneumomediastinum, the emergency physician transferred the patient to a tertiary care center. He was ultimately placed on comfort care and died several days later.

The intensivist called the emergency department medical director with a number of concerns. From his perspective, of course, it had been a simple intubation. So why did the emergency physician bungle the job?

Analysis

Among the challenges of practicing emergency medicine, along with night, weekend, and holiday shifts and bursts of chaos, is the huge bag of tricks that the emergency physician must carry. But within that bag of tricks, arguably the most important skill is *the ability to manage a difficult airway immediately*—especially when no anesthesiology back-up is available. As the case above demonstrates, however, having an anesthesiologist on deck is not always the solution.

The emergency physician had no difficulty in identifying the patient as a candidate for immediate intubation. He stated that even before the patient arrived, based upon the emergency medical services call, he had opened the crash cart and prepared the laryngoscope and tubes. When the patient vigorously fought the procedure, the physician ordered a dose of lorazepam—to no avail. He could not view the cords and made blind attempts to pass the tube. He ordered more lorazepam, which still did not help. Then the anesthesiologist arrived.

The obvious question is why the emergency physician did not do a rapid-sequence intubation (RSI). The physician stated that RSI had not been part of his training, and he had always been warned about the dangers of paralyzing awake patients.

Rapid-sequence intubation has evolved into a standard of care in emergency medicine, as most readers of this book are aware. This case illustrates its value perfectly. The old techniques of using "plain bruticane" or sequential doses of benzodiazepines to facilitate intubation have fallen by the wayside for good reason. But some emergency physicians have not yet become comfortable with RSI, and many emergency departments still encounter resistance from the anesthesiology department to creating RSI protocols. When the appropriate patient selection criteria are followed, the right medications are used, and an adequate back-up plan is in place, RSI is the safest, easiest method to ensure placement of an airway.

Numerous excellent national courses teach the management of difficult airways and include extensive training in all aspects of the RSI technique. They include hands-on training in the use of a number of adjuncts to airway control, such as cricothyroidotomy techniques. Such a course should be on the mandatory to-do list for any emergency physician who does not already possess extensive RSI experience or was not formally trained in RSI.

Teaching Points

1. RSI is a first-line option for the awake patient who requires intubation—not a last-ditch attempt.

2. Emergency physicians who are not comfortable with RSI should take one of the nationally recognized courses in management of the difficult airway.

3. Emergency departments should develop protocols for the use of RSI and also should have on hand several types of airway adjuncts (e.g., Combitubes, laryngeal mask airways, and lighted stylettes) in the event that an endotracheal tube cannot be placed.

68
To Tube or Not to Tube

During a lunch break, a 56-year-old teacher with a history of hypertension developed a severe headache accompanied by nausea and left-sided weakness. On arrival at the emergency department she was responsive only to painful stimuli, with no spontaneous movement of the left side. The emergency physician immediately suspected a major cerebrovascular catastrophe and, while arranging for air ambulance transport to the nearest facility with neurosurgical capacity, sent the patient to radiology for a CT scan of the head. On the CT table the patient had a seizure and vomited. A code was called, and the patient was intubated with some difficulty in the CT suite. CT demonstrated a large intracerebral hemorrhage.

The patient was transferred and taken to surgery, where blood was evacuated and bleeding controlled. She had a reasonable recovery, although her course was complicated by aspiration pneumonia and acute respiratory distress syndrome.

The director of radiology complained to the hospital administration that a comatose patient was sent for CT without being intubated. The emergency physician initially responded that in his view the patient did not need intubation before the CT because her airway was fine and her oxygen saturation excellent. In retrospect he agreed that he would never let a similar patient leave the emergency department without first controlling the airway.

Analysis

Endotracheal intubation not only provides a definitive airway for ventilation but also offers protection against the aspiration of regurgitated gastric contents or pooled saliva. The patient had lost the ability to protect her airway. It was perfectly predictable that her airway would only worsen over the short term because of the progression of the insult to the central nervous system. The best place for intubation is the controlled setting of the emergency department—not the CT suite.

The physician also reported that he did not intubate the patient before sending her to CT because she still had good muscle tone and was biting on the oral airway. He feared that her struggles during intubation would increase intracranial pressure. The answer to this dilemma, of course, is to use rapid sequence induction (RSI), which is the standard of care in emergency departments across the country—for good reason. Any emergency physician not yet familiar with RSI should take one of the excellent courses now available across the county in the management of difficult airways.

Teaching Points

1. Patients who need airway protection, such as patients who are comatose or severely obtunded for whatever reason, are candidates for preemptive intubation before leaving the emergency department for procedures or transfer.

2. Rapid sequence intubation techniques must be in the armamentarium of all emergency physicians.

3. Emergency departments that do not yet have RSI protocols need to develop them.

Case 69
The Worst Possible Scenario

A 10-year-old boy was riding unrestrained in the back of the family station wagon when it was struck broadside by a pick-up truck. He arrived in the emergency department with a laceration on the parietal scalp. He was awake but confused and was alternately drowsy and agitated. The emergency physician wanted to obtain a CT as quickly as possible, but because the boy was unable to cooperate or hold still, the physician decided to paralyze and intubate him to allow an optimal study. The patient was given an intravenous dose of succinylcholine and intubated. He was not pretreated with atropine. Before he could be taken to the radiology department, however, he began moving again and a second dose of succinylcholine was administered. He then left for the CT suite accompanied by a nurse. During the scan, he began thrashing. The nurse called the emergency department and was told to administer a third dose of succinylcholine.

After the scan was completed and the patient was wheeled back to the emergency department, he was noted to be bradycardic with a heart rate of less than 30 beats/min. His blood pressure was too low to measure.

Despite the use of atropine followed by vasopressors, the patient never regained adequate circulation and was pronounced dead in the emergency department.

His CT scan had been negative. An autopsy revealed no signs of internal trauma. The cause of death was listed as an untoward medication reaction.

Analysis

Few things are more tragic than the iatrogenic death of a child. Physicians who regularly use succinylcholine to facilitate intubations quickly grow fond of it. But appreciation must not grow into complacency. In general, when rapid sequence intubation is indicated in a child and succinylcholine is to be the paralytic agent, pretreatment with atropine is required. Because the cardiovascular system of children appears to be particularly sensitive to the depressant effects of succinylcholine, it should be used only with great caution. Repeat doses of succinylcholine should be avoided in children. If sedation is needed, other agents should be used.

Teaching Points

1. Any emergency department using succinylcholine must have a sound protocol in place to ensure that all emergency physicians are intimately familiar with the complications.

2. Never use succinylcholine for sedation. Safer alternatives include nondepolarizing agents with longer half-lives, such as vecuronium, or sedating agents, such as benzodiazepines, ditrovan, and etomidate.

3. Always pretreat children with atropine before administering succinylcholine, and avoid repeat doses.

Case 70
Chaos in a Small Space

A 75-year-old man was cutting down trees with his nephew when a dead branch broke off and struck him on the head, knocking him unconscious. His nephew placed him in the back of their pick-up truck, wrapped up in a tarp, and drove to a small rural hospital about 10 miles away. On arrival the patient—a previously healthy man—was awake but confused and agitated. He had a large scalp laceration and kept trying to get up from the stretcher. The triage nurse placed him in a rigid cervical collar, which he did not tolerate well. He became verbally abusive to the staff and refused to leave the collar in place.

The emergency physician on duty examined the patient. Rather than order a CT for a patient who may well have an intracranial bleed and require a neurosurgeon, he called the helicopter air ambulance and trauma center to arrange rapid transport. He gave the patient 1 mg of lorazepam intramuscularly to settle him down. By the time the helicopter arrived about 20 minutes later, the patient was unconscious and posturing. The emergency physician called the trauma center to advise them of the patient's deteriorating condition. Just before loading the patient on the helicopter, the emergency physician hung a bag of mannitol at the trauma surgeon's suggestion.

Ten minutes later, en route to the trauma center, the patient vomited and his breathing became labored. Multiple attempts by the flight crew to intubate the patient were unsuccessful, and on arrival the patient was bradycardic, pulseless, and apneic. Resuscitation efforts were unsuccessful. Autopsy revealed a large subdural hematoma with tentorial herniation.

The trauma center declared that a COBRA/EMTLA violation had been committed by the rural hospital because the patient's airway had not been secured, and his cervical spine had not been properly evaluated. Therefore, they contended that the patient was not adequately stabilized for the transfer. Appeals by the hospital and physician were to no avail; fines were levied against both.

Analysis

One of the keys to the successful practice of emergency medicine is the anticipation of disasters. The inability to control an airway is surely a catastrophe that must be avoided whenever possible. The emergency physician correctly assumed that the patient would need neurosurgical intervention. His decision to prioritize transport over obtaining a CT was absolutely correct. By the same logic, however, he should have realized that the patient would become less and less able to protect his own airway. Urgent intubation in the back of a helicopter is a daunting task in the best of hands. A rapid sequence intubation (RSI) before transport would have protected the patient's airway and allowed use of adequate sedation or long-acting paralytics to minimize the likelihood that the patient would worsen his injuries through excessive movement.

RSI also would have allowed the physician to keep the patient's neck more safely immobilized. Was cervical-spine clearance necessary before the patient left the rural emergency department, as the trauma center contended? Sometimes complete clearance—which in some cases requires a CT scan—is simply not feasible before transport. But with the patient adequately sedated and intubated and on a long board with the neck secured, transport without neck films beyond perhaps a simple x-ray would have been perfectly defensible on logistic and safety grounds.

Teaching Points

1. In patients with significant head injuries—especially those who are agitated, combative, or becoming rapidly obtunded—RSI should be done early.

2. RSI not only protects the patient against airway compromise but also allows safer sedation to facilitate the performance of studies and transfer.

3. Never let a patient at risk for airway compromise leave the department unintubated.

Chapter 13

Case 71
The Patient's Perceptions

A 46-year-old nurse manager was walking down a corridor in the hospital when she developed a sudden, brief sense of imbalance and lightheadedness, the like of which she had never experienced before. After a few moments, she went about her business, but the sensation returned an hour later, and this time lasted several minutes. At the end of her shift she came to the emergency department and told her story to the charge nurse, who encouraged her to be checked out.

The emergency physician knew the patient well, having taught pediatric advanced life support courses with her. Although a little overweight, she was otherwise healthy. The patient herself suggested that the problem was probably labyrinthitis. A brief neurologic exam was normal. The symptoms could not be replicated by changes in head position. The EKG was normal. She again suggested a diagnosis of labyrinthitis. Although the clinical picture did not fit well with the peripheral vertigo symptoms of labyrinthitis, the physician agreed that it was a likely possibility and discharged her with a prescription for meclizine and instructions to seek further evaluation later that week.

In bed that night a gagging sound awakened the patient's husband. She was unresponsive and had no pulse. He called 911 and began CPR. Despite extensive resuscitation efforts by the emergency medical technicians and then the emergency department personnel, she did not regain circulation and was pronounced dead. The autopsy was completely normal. The cause of death was listed as "probable cardiac arrhythmia."

Analysis

It is painful for physicians to feel that they may have prevented the death of a friend under their care, despite reassurances from colleagues that they would have done nothing different in the same situation.

Be that as it may, there are lessons to be learned. Clearly, both the emergency physician and the patient herself wanted the problem to be something simple and self-limiting. As the physician later reported, when he first walked in the room and said hello, the patient's response was to apologize for bothering him: "I know this is nothing. Can I go now?" On some level the physician may have agreed with her and thereby ignored some of the darker possibilities that may have explained her symptoms.

This is not to say that every patient with nonspecific dizziness requires a million-dollar work-up. Before deciding how far to go, the physician must begin with a careful attempt to categorize the symptoms. In general, dizzy spells mean one of three things: (1) the hallucination of motion, as in vertigo; (2) a sense of lightheadedness, as in faintness; or (3) a sense of disequilibrium. Although these symptoms are often so tightly woven together that it may be impossible to separate them completely, the clinician must tease them apart as delicately as possible—for each engages a different differential diagnosis. One trick many clinicians use is to ask for a description of the symptom excluding the word *dizziness*.

If the symptom is actually vertigo, the physician must differentiate between the abrupt, transient, head position-related symptoms of peripheral vertigo and the more subacute and vague sensations of central vertigo.

True disequilibrium, on the other hand, is usually a more chronic condition related to diminished sensory input secondary to neuropathies and the aging process.

Dizziness that is actually transient lightheadedness—i.e., presyncope—is most often related to a decrease in central circulation caused by neurovascular, cardiovascular, or cerebrovascular conditions.

In retrospect, the nurse was having presyncopal episodes. It is possible that if the physician had questioned her more forcefully about the exact nature of the symptom and had disengaged his subjective desire for a good outcome, the true differential diagnosis would have come into better focus. The thought that he might have saved her life will always haunt the physician.

Teaching Points

1. Always carefully distinguish the characteristics of "dizziness" by asking the patient to describe the event in other terms. The extra minutes are necessary and worth the effort.

2. Be especially vigilant against overoptimism when dealing with patient well known to you or with family members.

3. If the dizzy spell is actually presyncope, always consider a possible cardiogenic cause and act accordingly. Appropriate action may involve admission for telemetry or outpatient Holter monitoring, depending on the patient's age, general condition, and presence of other risk factors.

Case 72
Tank Them Up

A 29-year-old man with a 5-year history of diabetes mellitus presented to the emergency department with the complaint of feeling weak and nauseated since the previous day. He reported vomiting approximately 10 times over the past 24 hours. The illness, he said, actually began about four days ago with nasal congestion and pain in both ears. He had not eaten since the previous night and had not taken his insulin that morning.

According to the triage note, he was a slender, tired-looking man. He was afebrile. His pulse rate was 105 beats/min, his blood pressure was 118/84 mmHg, and his respiratory rate was 24 breaths/min. On examination, the tympanic membranes were dull and red bilaterally, and his mucous membranes were quite dry. His abdomen was benign, and his chest was clear. The emergency physician also wrote that the odor of ketone was detectable from across the room.

She initiated fluid therapy and ordered blood work, and shortly afterward the presumptive diagnosis of diabetic ketoacidosis was confirmed by the lab. Serum and urine were positive for ketones, the glucose level was 444 mg/dl, the sodium level was 131 mEq/L, and the bicarbonate level was 18 mEq/L. Blood urea nitrogen and creatinine were mildly elevated, but the complete blood count was normal. The emergency physician asked the physician on call for the number of the patient's primary provider to discuss admission. The on-call admitting doctor, however, suggested that the emergency physician try to treat the patient in the emergency department and determine whether he was dischargable. The emergency physician agreed—somewhat reluctantly, she said later. She ordered 10 units of regular insulin intravenously, along with 3 liters of normal saline to be given over 3 hours.

Meanwhile, a new emergency physician came on duty. After the fluids were infused, he ordered a repeat set of lab tests. The glucose level was improved at 355 mg/dl, but the bicarbonate level had only decreased by 1 to 17 mEq/L. The patient looked good, however, and reported feeling much better. After proving that he could hold down some ginger ale, the patient was discharged with a prescription for amoxicillin to treat bilateral otitis media.

Once home, the patient was unable to keep fluids down. After a night's valiant effort of hoping the symptoms would improve spontaneously— capped by a faint as he walked to the bathroom that morning—the young man returned to the emergency department, with orthostatic changes and a laceration on his forehead. He was admitted and spent 4 days as an inpatient.

His primary physician called the medical director to ask why the patient was not admitted on his first visit.

Analysis

All physicians face mounting pressure from third-party payors and utilization review coordinators to avoid admitting patients whenever possible. Acute illnesses such as diabetic ketoacidosis (DKA)—once clear-cut tickets for admission—are now believed to be potentially treatable in the ambulatory setting. In many cases, this attitude is quite reasonable. It is far from bad medicine to consider treating patients with mild DKA in the emergency department with fluid replacement and insulin, assuming that the physician formulates appropriate decision-making criteria so that if the patient fails ambulatory treatment, an admission will follow. Such decision-making criteria may include repeat lab studies, as in this case. The problem, of course, is that the second set of lab tests showed a worsening bicarbonate level, suggesting that the patient was still too sick to go home, despite his subjective improvement. If a clinician orders labs tests to help make disposition decisions, they must be used as such.

When we think of how this problem might have been avoided, several issues are worth noting. The first physician felt from the onset that the patient needed admission and that the doctor covering for the patient's primary care provider was procrastinating. She would have been within her rights to disagree—a politically painful but sometimes necessary step when an on-call physician tries to avoid an admission. One point is certain: every time a patient is passed from one physician to another at shift change, the chance of making a mistake increases. There is an often observed tendency for the second (or third) emergency physician not to feel as great a sense of ownership toward the patient as the initial physician does. In this case, the second emergency physician—who actually discharged the patient—stated that all he heard from the first emergency physician was that the patient was "ready to roll" after a little more fluid and a quick recheck. There was only a verbal sign-off—no exchange of notes or writing down of information.

The lessons are clear. When relegating the care of a patient whose disposition is in doubt, make sure that the relieving physician understands the issues at stake. Jotting down crucial points on a 3-by-5 card is time well spent. Receiving physicians—no matter how busy the emergency department may be with new patients—must assume complete ownership, taking nothing for granted.

One also must wonder why an antiemetic agent was not prescribed for the patient at the time of discharge.

Teaching Points

1. Be wary of shift-change time when relegating patients who have doubtful dispositions.

2. Give notes on complex patients to relieving physicians.

3. Emergency physicians must take full ownership of patients passed to them at shift changes.

4. Make every effort to complete a disposition rather than to pass the patient to the next physician. Force the issue of admission if you feel that it is needed.

5. If follow-up lab tests are ordered, the results must be used appropriately. Overlooked results are worse than no results at all.

6. Patients with diabetic ketoacidosis may be treated and released after prolonged emergency department hydration and insulin therapy, but only if all clinical factors show definite improvement.

Case 73
Give Them a Break

An 83-year-old woman came to the emergency department after 5 days of cough and increasing shortness of breath. Two days earlier she had called her family doctor, who telephoned a prescription for ciprofloxacin. The antibiotic did not improve her symptoms. Along with a history of hypertension and several minor cerebrovascular accidents, the patient had been diagnosed a few years previously with mild chronic obstructive pulmonary disease, for which she occasionally used a combination of bronchodilators by metered-dose inhaler. The inhaler had not helped much recently.

On arrival at the emergency department her temperature was 99.7° F, her blood pressure 160/90 mm Hg, and her respiratory rate was 28 breaths/min. Initial oxygen saturation was recorded on the chart. The emergency physician examined the patient and found her reasonably comfortable, quite alert, and, as his note recorded, "feisty." Chest auscultation revealed generally diminished breath sounds, especially at the right base, with some diffuse expiratory wheezing. She had no signs of congestive failure. Because her skin felt hot, the emergency physician asked for a rectal temperature, which demonstrated a fever of 101.2° F. The emergency physician ordered lab tests, x-rays, acetaminophen, and a treatment of nebulized albuteral. The chest x-ray showed pneumonia in the right lower lobe. The white blood cell count was 15,000/μL with 92% granulocytes and 2% band forms. Serum chemistries were normal.

After two bronchodilator treatments and an antipyretic, the patient seemed more comfortable and her fever had subsided. She took a meal without problems and firmly requested to be discharged. The emergency physician, as he later stated, agreed reluctantly. She was given a dose of clarithromycin in the emergency department and a prescription for the same drug as well as for a tapered course of prednisone. She was sent home with instructions to see her primary physician in 1–2 days. She lived alone. No discharge oxygen saturation was recorded in the chart.

Late that evening the patient's daughter found her lying in bed seeming quite short of breath. The daughter decided to take her back to the emergency department the next morning, but during the night the patient stumbled while walking to the bathroom and landed on her left hip. She was transported by emergency medical services to the emergency department, where her initial oxygen saturation was 89% and x-rays demonstrated a hip fracture.

Although the patient recovered well from the pneumonia and subsequent orthopedic surgery, her daughter filed a formal complaint with the state health department about the emergency physician's decision to discharge her mother after the first emergency department visit.

Analysis

One of the difficulties in reviewing cases is that the reviewer did not see the patient. The first emergency physician made the case that the patient looked well on the first day—sprightly and full of vinegar. But the likelihood of a "bounce-back" was high. She had already failed a course of outpatient ciprofloxacin (the choice of antibiotic was not ideal for community-acquired pneumonia). Her age, the elevated white blood cell count, the fever, the fact that she lived alone—all constituted a good case for admission.

On the other hand, a physician cannot force a competent adult into the hospital against her will. The emergency physician said that he spent at least 5 minutes arguing in favor of admission but she was determined to go home. The problem is that he mentions none of this interchange in the chart.

The special reviewer sent by the state health department cited the lack of documentation as a major clinical deficit. If the physician truly believed that the patient needed admission, why did not he not have her sign out against medical advice? Why did he not bring the patient's primary physician into the loop, at least by arranging a definite follow-up visit on the next day, instead of leaving the follow-up plan vague and patient-driven? Only with the help of an attorney, paid by himself, did the physician avoid a citation and settled instead for a hundred percent chart review for a 6-month period.

The lesson is obvious. If an emergency physician discharges a patient at high risk for complications, the rationale needs to be well documented. Patient reluctance also needs to be documented—by an against-medical-advice form, if necessary. Indeed, sometimes the act of asking the patient to sign the form can underline the seriousness of a situation and help to convince the patient to take the safer course. If the patient still insists on leaving, at least it is recorded in black and white that the clinician did all that he or she could have done. It remains a truism: *if it wasn't written, it wasn't done.*

One positive aspect of the case deserves discussion. The physician did not trust the oral temperature. Oral temperatures are far less reliable than rectal temperatures. If the presence of a fever would make a difference in diagnosis, treatment, or disposition and if the oral temperature is normal, hyperthermia must be ruled out rectally. The same is true for tympanic temperatures, which have generally been found to be less reliable than oral measurements.[1,2]

Teaching Points

1. If a borderline candidate for admission is not admitted, the emergency physician must document his or her rationale for discharge.

2. For a patient who clearly needs but refuses admission, the physician must document the refusal, using an against-medical-advice form if necessary.

3. All relevant clinical information for patients, such as the pulse oximetry in patients with lung disease or infections, should be documented.

4. Do not rely on tympanic or oral temperature measurement in patients who may have a fever and for whom the presence of fever may alter diagnosis, treatment, or disposition.

References

1. Hooker EA, et al: Screening for fever in an adult emergency department: Oral vs. tympanic thermometry. South Med J 89:230, 1996.
2. Petersen-Smith A, et al: Comparison of aural infrared with traditional rectal temperatures in children from birth to age three years. J Pediatr 125:83, 1994.

Case 74
A Faint

A 79-year-old woman was brought to the emergency department by her niece. They had just finished lunch at a restaurant when the patient became pale and slumped forward over the table. She returned to herself in little more than a minute, but the niece decided that a visit to the emergency department was appropriate.

This generally healthy woman had no previous episodes of syncope and no major history of cardiac disease. She was taking medications for hypertension and hypercholesterolemia, but she had no history, of diabetes or strokes. Her vital signs were perfectly normal, as was a thorough physical examination. The emergency physician ordered routine lab tests, an EKG and a CT scan of the head. All were normal, as documented in the physician's comprehensive note. The physician discharged the patient with a diagnosis of "probable vasovagal syncope, post-prandial" and instructed her to see her regular doctor in 3 to 5 days for further evaluation.

Unfortunately, the patient collapsed at home on the following day. She was brought to the emergency department and pronounced dead shortly thereafter. The case came to review as an unexpected revisit with complications within less than 72 hours. The family contacted an attorney.

Analysis

Syncope, especially among the elderly, is not among the favorite chief complaints of most emergency physicians. The required work-up is extensive yet seldom definitive. The differential diagnosis contains some really bad actors (e.g., malignant cardiac arrthymias) that usually lurk out of diagnostic reach in the emergency department. For this reason, many physicians consider admission to be the safest course for unexplained syncope in middle-aged or elderly patients. Yet many admitting physicians fight against the emergency physician's desire to have the patient observed in a safe, monitored environment.

The emergency physician often has to battle for an appropriate disposition.

The main overall cause of syncope is the so-called vasovagal or reflex vasomotor hypotension. But this benign entity is almost always a diagnosis of circumstance and exclusion. Furthermore, with age the frequency of more serious entities rises, making it less safe to assume that a vasovagal episode was the culprit. Therefore, as a general rule, unless the circumstances definitely point toward a vasovagal event in a patient with a clear-cut history of similar events, older patients with new-onset syncope ideally should be admitted for further evaluation. This patient was elderly, had cardiac risk factors, and lacked a known history of fainting spells. The probability of cardiac syncope was high enough to justify consideration for admission, or, at an absolute minimum, contact with a follow-up physician to arrange definitive evaluation in a timely fashion.

Despite the excellent documentation otherwise found in the chart, the emergency physician left the follow-up arrangements uncertain and solely patient-driven. This disposition in an elderly patient with syncope puts both patient and physician at the mercy of Murphy's law.

Teaching Points

1. Emergency physicians should have a low threshold for admitting middle-aged and elderly patients with new-onset syncope.

2. When patients are discharged with a diagnosis of syncope of uncertain etiology, make follow-up arrangements as definitive and timely as possible.

Case 75
Breathless

A 65-year-old man with chronic obstructive pulmonary disease (COPD) presented to the emergency department with a 2-day history of worsening cough and exertional dyspnea. He also told the triage nurse that he had experienced chest pain, although this symptom was not further characterized in the nurse's note. Although his lips were cyanotic, he was alert and oriented, with a heart rate of 103 beats/min, a respiratory rate of 25 breaths/min, and an oxygen saturation of 84% on room air. He was afebrile. Routine medications at home included bronchodilator metered-dose inhalers, prednisone, metoprolol, and a long-acting nitrate. He had had numerous admissions to the same emergency department in recent years for exacerbations of COPD, which usually did not require admission. The patient reported that his family doctor was in the process of getting him oxygen at home. He was immediately placed on oxygen by nasal cannula at 3 L/min, and his pulse oximetry rose and stabilized at 94%.

By the time the emergency physician examined him, the patient was much more comfortable. The physician's note, in fact, described him as "jovial and alert." His breath sounds, however, were distant, and expiratory wheezes were present diffusely. The emergency physician ordered several nebulized bronchodilator treatments and an intravenous dose of solumedrol. The physician's note contained no reference to chest pain.

Given the patient's dramatic response to oxygen and his plans to have oxygen at home, the emergency physician called the respiratory technician to help make arrangements for delivery of an oxygen tank. The necessary tank and equipment were to be delivered to the patient's home later that evening.

Meanwhile, the patient continued to look and feel good. After a 3-hour stay in the emergency department he was discharged. The emergency physician did not order an EKG and did not make formal contact with the family doctor.

About 2 hours after discharge, while still waiting for the oxygen tank to be delivered, the patient complained to his wife of crushing chest pain. She called 911, but when the medics arrived, the patient was bradycardic, pulseless, and having agonal respirations. He was coded en route to the emergency department, where he was pronounced dead half an hour after arrival.

Analysis

At one time or another, most emergency physicians have had the not entirely pleasant experience of noticing a piece of information in a nursing note that they did not get from the patient, and that the nurse did not verbally bring to their attention. Sometimes it is an important piece of information. Usually, the physician notices the discrepancy before the patient leaves the emergency department. But once in a while, the patient has already gone home.

The physician admitted that he would have ordered an EKG and, even if it were normal, probably would not have discharged the patient, given his hypoxia and cardiac risk factors in general. "But I was so focused on getting this guy set up with home oxygen, because he clearly had needed it for a while and his family doctor had dropped the ball." The emergency physician further stated that, in fact, he believed that he had asked the man about chest pain and that he denied it. But the emergency physician was not absolutely certain; in any case, he left no record on the chart.

This case tragically emphasizes the importance of scanning the nursing note. Emergency physicians must accept the fact that, for various reasons, a nurse may not transmit a piece of information verbally. They may forget, they may go off shift, they may be distracted, or they may be in a different area of the emergency department. They have every right to believe that the physician will read the note. The emergency physician must not assume that a nurse will otherwise guide him to every important fact. This case also illustrates another issue. In general, home oxygen therapy is best arranged by the primary physician, or at least in close cooperation with the doctor who has a long-term rela-tionship with the patient. The primary physician is the only one posi-tioned to handle the multiple follow-up issues, including questions about reimbursement by third-party carriers.

In this case, if the emergency physician had either discovered and characterized the complaint of chest pain, or if he had simply not made the decision to obtain home oxygen, the patient would have been admitted, and his death and the subsequent litigation might have been avoided.

Teaching Points

1. Always read the nursing notes.

2. In patients who are in any way at risk for cardiac ischemia, despite the presence of an apparently unrelated chief complaint, do a review of systems that includes asking about chest pain.

3. Make arrangements for home oxygen therapy only in concert with the primary physician, or leave the decision about such therapy to him or her alone.

Case 76
Big Bad Wolf

A scruffy looking young man with a paint-spattered beard staggered unsteadily up to the triage desk, stating that he had been "huffing" paint fumes and did not feel well. The triage nurse promptly led him to the treatment area. She helped him onto a stretcher and took his vital signs. They were normal, but according to her note, his speech was slurred and he was "not highly oriented." She put him on a monitor, pulled up the side rails and informed the emergency physician of his presence.

It was a busy day. The emergency physician thanked her for the information and returned to a chart rack full of patients yet to be seen.

Twenty minutes later a different nurse noticed the patient walking toward the ambulance entrance. She stopped and questioned him. He said that he felt better and needed to leave. She managed to herd him back into the room, then went to tell the physician, who was in the process of repairing a laceration. The physician told her that if the patient was ambulatory and wanted to leave, have him sign out against medical advice. The patient did so, though his signature on the form was nothing more than an irregular line.

The next day, a peer reviewer flagged this chart, feeling that the patient deserved further evaluation before being allowed to sign out against medical advice. The telephone number left by the patient was not in service, and he was lost to follow-up.

Analysis

This case illustrates several issues. First is that life in the emergency department does not follow a straight line. Certain patients demand immediate attention, regardless of how many others are at the front of the line. No emergency physician would argue against this principle when life or death problems are involved. But what about this patient? Should the emergency physician have broken off what he was doing and at least briefly checked the patient before letting him depart?

The chronically troublesome issue is determining what constitutes patient competence. To sign out against medical advice implies that a patient can reasonably comprehend the advice—that he or she has sufficient judgment to understand the possible negative consequences of the decision to leave. This particular patient may well have come down enough from his "high" to assume responsibility for his decision. On the other hand, we cannot know—and neither could the emergency physician.

We should not make a hard and fast rule that every patient desiring to sign out against medical advice needs the physician's intervention. Such a policy makes no sense, for example, when a patient with a minor sprain tires of waiting after 4 hours. Many patients who sign out against medical advice fit into this category. But when the patient is intoxicated or has a potentially life-threatening symptom, wise practice warrants that the physician become immediately involved, at least until he or she determines whether a critical situation exits.

If an intoxicated patient who is clearly not able to make rational decisions about his or her immediate well-being wants to leave, current risk-management teaching leans toward a course in which the emergency physician should consider chemical restraint, if necessary, to allow for patient safety and further evaluation. Such decisions must be individualized, taking all factors—including the safety of staff—into consideration.

Teaching Points

1. Emergency physicians should make every effort to evaluate promptly patients who desire to sign out against medical advice and who are intoxicated or have potentially life-threatening symptoms, such as chest pain or severe headache.

2. Good public relations dictate that the physician see *all* patients who want to leave against medical advice, although this is not always practical.

3. Obviously intoxicated patients who are unable to make rational judgments and desire to leave are potential candidates for chemical restraint.

Case 77
Absconding

A 35-year-old man presented to the emergency department one evening, moderately intoxicated and asking for help in finding a detoxification facility. His home was in a city about 150 miles away. He was visiting a friend and had nowhere to go. He had no previous history of contact with an alcohol rehabilitation program. The emergency physician believed that he was sincere about wanting help and not simply looking for a bed and a meal. The emergency physician examined the patient. He showed no signs of alcohol withdrawal, and his blood alcohol level was 150 mg/dl. The social worker came to the emergency department at the physician's request and began searching for a facility that might accept the patient.

The emergency department was becoming busy. To free up a room, the patient was taken to the quiet room to await the outcome of his transfer arrangements to a detoxification and rehabilitation facility.

Meanwhile, another intoxicated patient had come into the emergency department for quite different reasons. He had suffered a scalp laceration after being struck by a beer bottle and wanted no further assistance. The emergency physician repaired his laceration and felt that he presented no danger to himself. A friend agreed to pick him up, and he was asked to wait in the quiet room until his ride came.

Half an hour later the emergency physician went to inform the first patient that a bed had been found for him at a nearby hospital. He discovered, however, that the quiet room was empty.

The first patient returned by ambulance several hours later. While running across the interstate highway following his new friend to a bar, he had been struck by a car. He had a severe head injury and was pronounced dead in the emergency department.

Several months later, the patient's family initiated a suit against the physician and the hospital on the grounds that they had failed to take reasonable precautions to secure the patient's safety. A jury verdict in favor of the man's family was ultimately overturned on appeal after great expense and emotional distress for everyone concerned.

Analysis

The debate generated by such a case centers on issues of personal responsibility and free will. Did the physician compromise the patient's safety by leaving him unsupervised with a potential drinking partner? Or did the patient simply make a choice of his own volition for which the physician and hospital bear no burden of guilt whatsoever? The answer surely lies somewhere between. Once the emergency physician decided to take the humanitarian step of trying to help the patient, extra responsibility was generated.

The emergency physician stated that he was unaware that the two men were put together, that the nurse made this arrangement without his knowledge, and that if he had known, he would not have condoned the arrangement. Be that as it may, it makes sense for emergency departments to segregate patients awaiting transfer from patients awaiting discharge. Such a policy probably would have prevented this unfortunate outcome.

Teaching Points

1. Always engage in worst-case thinking with regard to the possibility of elopement when patients are awaiting disposition or transfer—especially for substance abuse or psychiatric reasons.

2. It is generally wiser to keep such patients under the best conditions of observation that the resources of a particular emergency department allow.

Case 78
It's Not Over Till the Clean Up Is Done

A 67-year-old woman, accompanied by her daughter, presented early Sunday morning with a nosebleed. The patient said that her nose had been bleeding on and off for several days. Yesterday, in fact, she had gone to an urgent care center where a physician staunched the bleeding by "burning it with something on a stick." She was fine all night, until a sneeze the next morning started the bleeding again.

On arrival in the emergency department, the woman's vital signs were normal. She had no history of a bleeding diathesis, was taking no anticoagulants, and had no previous problems with significant epistaxis. The patient denied nasal trauma.

The emergency physician examined the patient and discovered several areas of oozing in the region of Kiesselbach's plexus on the anterior septum. Rather than attempt another cauterization and risk damaging the septum, the emergency physician decided to apply phenylephrine and place a packing in the nostril.

Packing went without incident. The emergency physician gave the patient a prescription for cephalexin to protect against the potential for infection related to the packing and said that he wanted to watch her for another half an hour before discharge. He then left the room.

Approximately ten minutes later a loud crash was heard from the patients' room. The patient's daughter, who had been sitting near the tray of bloody gauze and instruments, had fainted, striking the Mayo stand, sending a tray of instruments flying, and receiving a gash to her cheek that required eight sutures. The entire contents of tray— including an emesis basis containing blood and phlegm—had landed on top of her.

A complaint to the administration soon followed. The hospital president personally called to speak with the patient and her daughter. Both commended the emergency department staff for its prompt care. They even complimented the physician's bedside manner and competence in dealing with the nosebleed. But both wondered why the physician had not been sensitive to the filthy Mayo stand left by the stretcher. He knew that they would be sitting next to it for half an hour, and it was not a busy day. The daughter felt sure that the stand had caused her to faint. She had already told the doctor that she was feeling a little woozy.

Analysis

Many physicians become so accustomed to gruesome sights that they sometimes forget the noxious impact that such things as blood, emesis, and phlegm can have on people not accustomed to them. Physicians also can become a bit spoiled by the fact that usually someone else will clean things up. But the few seconds that it takes to push a tray of soiled material away from the bedside or to cover a mess with a towel is time wisely invested. It can spare a patient or family member unnecessary distress and is the mark of a seasoned and sensitive clinician.

Every emergency physician has had (or will have) the experience of a family member, friend, or loved one "passing out" by the bedside, most often during procedures that they wanted to watch. There is nothing wrong with letting people watch, but some caveats are in order. Consider limiting the number of bystanders to one or two. Ask them if they have ever fainted in a medical setting before, and if they have, they should not stay. They should sit and not stand. They should be warned to lower their heads or leave the room if they begin to feel lightheaded, warm, sweaty, uneasy, or nauseated. And the emergency physician should ask periodically if they are feeling all right. Better to have the mom whose face is turning pale and clammy leave than to pick her up from the floor. Usually, bystanders do not argue.

Teaching Points

1. Emergency physicians should make an effort not to expose patients and family members to postprocedural gore longer than necessary.

2. Emergency physicians should not hesitate to remove or cover a tray themselves, if the need arises.

3. Family members or bystanders should be limited in number and screened for a history of syncope. They should sit, not stand, and should be warned of the symptoms of an impending faint.

Case 79
Moats in the Eye

An ophthalmologist called the director of the emergency department one morning to complain about the way a patient was cared for the day before. In fact, the patient was sitting in the ophthalmologist's examining chair with a metallic foreign body imbedded in his left cornea—an injury missed by the emergency physician on the previous night. But what had spurred the ophthalmologist to make the call was the bottle of tetracaine topical anesthetic that the patient had used to self-medicate his pain through the night. The patient said that the emergency physician had given it to him. The ophthalmologist said that the foreign body was obvious and should not have been missed in the first place, and that home medication with tetracaine was contraindicated in general. He wanted to warn the emergency department director that a formal complaint against the emergency physician would be aggressively pursued.

The case was investigated. The emergency department log showed that it had been an extremely busy Monday evening. The chart stated that the emergency physician had checked the man's visual acuity and noted that diffuse conjunctival injection and some purulent material were present at the medial canthus, that the pupil was symmetric and responsive to light, that the anterior chamber was clear, and that no foreign bodies were obvious. In addition, the emergency physician noted that the man had a recent "cold" and that his son was out of school for "pink eye." The discharge noted an impression of "conjunctivitis." There was no mention of giving the patient tetracaine to take home. There was also no mention of using fluorescein or of a slit lamp examination.

Upon questioning, the emergency physician denied having given the man a topical anesthetic agent to use at home but reported that he had left a bottle of tetracaine on the stand next to the patient after his evaluation. As for not looking at the eye more carefully for foreign bodies with fluorescein dye or slit lamp, he said that the history of pink eye in one of this children and the presence of purulent discharge must have misled him. Ordinarily he always checked for foreign bodies, but it was a busy day. He had not asked the patient if he might have been doing an activity—such as grinding metal or working under a car—that might have sent a foreign body into the eye.

Analysis

The standard emergency department acute eye exam in adults must—at a minimum—include visual acuity, assessment for photophobia, pupillary light reactivity, and clarity of the anterior chamber, and a careful visual search for foreign bodies on the globe and under both lids. A fluorescein dye exam is always a wise investment of time, and if doubt remains, a general exam with the slit lamp is a good idea. Any acute eye discomfort in adults should be considered the result of a foreign body or a corneal abrasion until proved otherwise. Patients with constant severe ocular pain and visual impairment also should receive tonometry. In children, the cause of an eye problem is more likely to be infectious; a fluorescein dye exam is also indicated if there is any question of an abrasion. In fact, any preverbal infant with unexplained crying should be evaluated for the presence of an occult corneal abrasion.

The emergency physician did not make the best decision when he chose to skip a fluorescein or slit lamp exam. Given the fact that most metallic foreign bodies on the cornea can be seen with a careful visual exam alone, it is likely that he had already made up his mind that the patient had a case of conjunctivitis and did not look further.

As for the tetracaine, there is little doubt that the patient simply borrowed it after the physician departed. Anything that we leave in the room can be "borrowed"—a problem that may occur more often than we think. Medication should not be left in the room alone with a patient. The urge to self-medicate may be too great. The risks of a patient using a topical anesthetic on the eye at home for prolonged periods include the potential for delayed healing, inadvertent reinjury, and failure to seek appropriate follow-up care.

Teaching Points

1. Always include a careful search for foreign bodies in patients with ocular pain.

2. Ophthalmologic topical anesthetics, because of their power to give dramatic pain relief and the fact that they are forbidden fruit, may find their way out of the department without the emergency physician's knowledge.

Case 80
The Tooth of the Matter

One of the staff neurologists called the medical director about a 30-year-old woman seen two days earlier in the emergency department. She had been referred to the neurologist for evaluation of possible trigeminal neuralgia and was currently in his office. The neurologist wanted the medical director to know that the woman began spontaneously draining pus from a dental abscess in one of her upper left molars. He was sending her across the street to see a dentist. The abscess was the source of her facial pain.

When the medical director spoke to the patient the next day, she told him that the emergency physician had looked in her mouth but had not touched her teeth. A conversation with the emergency physician confirmed her report.

Analysis

Facial pain is a common presenting complaint to emergency departments with a differential that includes Bell's palsy, trigeminal neuralgia, herpes zoster, temporomandibular joint syndrome, cardiac disease, salivary gland calculi, parotitis, and dental problems. One of the best ways to assess dental problems, of course, is to percuss each tooth with an object such as a tooth blade and to palpate the alveolar-buccal gutter with a gloved finger. If that had been done, the correct diagnosis probably would have been discovered and an unnecessary visit to the neurologist avoided.

Teaching Points

1. Careful examination of the teeth is warranted in all patients with facial pain.

2. The pain of trigeminal neuralgia tends to be lancinating and intermittent, whereas the pain of a dental infection is more constant and worsened by percussion of the involved tooth.

Case 81
But Does It Fit the Picture?

A 49-year-old homeless man came to the emergency department complaining of a toothache with right lower jaw pain and swelling for 2 weeks. He had no difficulty in breathing or swallowing and denied any fever, although he was not a good historian. Examination revealed some facial asymmetry due to swelling near the angle of the mandible on the right. His dentition was poor, with numerous missing teeth and marked decay of the rest. None of the remaining teeth appeared tender to percussion with a tongue blade.

The emergency physician diagnosed a dental abscess and discharged the patient with prescriptions for penicillin and acetaminophen with codeine. There were no specific follow-up instructions beyond recommending a visit with a dentist.

Five weeks later one of the staff otolaryngologists called the emergency department director to inform her that an emergency physician had made a poor call with this patient. A dental clinic had referred the patient to his office a few days before, and he had just confirmed the diagnosis of pharyngeal carcinoma. The month of lost time had made the prognosis grimmer than it might have been. The patient had not been able to locate a private dentist because of his lack of health insurance.

Analysis

Many emergency physicians have had fairly limited exposure to dental problems in their training and experience. Nonetheless, they must routinely deal with patients who have severe dental pain secondary to periapical and periodontal abscesses and post-extraction alveolitis (dry socket). The conditions are usually acute and often accompanied by visible external swelling. Characteristically, the involved tooth is exquisitely sensitive. Because odontogenic infections can spread, the emergency physician must look for signs of potentially dangerous, airway-threatening, deep-space infections, such as Ludwig's angina (bilateral submandibular and sublingual cellulitis). Dental infections also can lead to the devastating complication of cavernous sinus thrombosis through retrograde spread up the ophthalmic veins.

The emergency physician said that he realized that the patient's presentation was "not a hundred percent classic" for a dental abscess, but it seemed reasonable to start there rather than to chase zebras. The patient's dentition was horrendous, and if you hear hoof beats, think horses.

That old adage, of course, is a good one, but only if one really hears hoof beats. This patient's lack of a tender tooth on exam, combined with the prolonged nonacute course, made it an *extremely* atypical dental infection—so atypical as to demand rethinking and referral rather than reflexive action.

Teaching Points

1. The differential diagnosis for progressive, subacute swelling of the face contains some bad actors, including perioral carcinomas. Patients with facial infections tend toward a more acute, toxic-appearing scenario.

2. When dealing with any condition that does not fit well into the usual pattern, make sure that the follow-up plan is as realistic and definite as possible.

Case 82
More than Meets the Eye

A 60-year-old retired man had been clearing and burning brush on his farm and came into the emergency department with swelling, redness, and itchiness of the right side of his face. He reported no previous history of similar symptoms. A large area of induration covered his left cheek and extended around the left eye, with marked periorbital puffiness. The eye was normal. The skin was mildly pink and not warm to the touch, and the patient was not febrile. Blisters were noted on the cheek and nose. The emergency physician felt comfortable that the patient did not have erysipilis or facial cellulites based on the clinical appearance. The patient wondered if he might have poison ivy. The emergency physician agreed that this was the most plausible diagnosis and discharged the man with a prescription for a course of tapered prednisone.

Over the next two days, the man developed more vesicular lesions in the affected area, along with increasing discomfort in the eye itself. He consulted with his internist, who made the diagnosis of shingles and commented negatively on the emergency physician's general lack of acumen. He referred the man to an ophthalmologist for treatment of zoster ophthalmicus. The man called a friend on the hospital board to complain.

Analysis

It would probably surprise no one that the first case of medical malpractice on record in English common law was generated when a second physician disparaged the care given by another physician for a hand injury (*Stratton v. Swanlond,* 1375). Be that as it may, the unilateral, dermatomal nature of the man's condition, along with the presence of a "blister," should have signaled something other than contact dermatitis to the emergency physician. The emergency physician said later that the diffuse skin changes and the periorbital puffiness misled him.

Teaching Points

1. Early shingles can present with only pain, but other more diffuse skin changes may be present as the conditions progress.

2. In facial zoster, the presence of lesions on the nose suggests involvement of the ophthalmic branch of the facial nerve and mandates ophthalmologic consultation.

Case 83
A Noxious Stimulus

A 29-year-old woman came to emergency department with the odor of alcohol on her breath after fainting at home. Although she was reasonably awake on arrival, the emergency department nurses noted that she entered a comatose state when her mother or significant other entered the treatment room. She also became comatose shortly after the emergency physician began to examine her. The nurse handed the emergency physician an ammonium capsule, which he broke and held under the patient's nose. She woke, began to yell, and tried to punch the doctor and nurse. When her aggressiveness subsided, the physician performed his exam and ordered routine lab tests. Her blood alcohol level was 290 mg/dl; other lab tests were normal.

After an observation period of 3½ hours, the patient was calm and cooperative. She had been under recent stress at work and home, and was not suicidal. She was not a regular consumer of alcohol in large quantities, as she had done earlier that day. Although the patient was not completely sober, the emergency physician believed that it was safe to accede to her request and allow her to go home with her family, who were clearly supportive and had good insight into the situation.

Nothing more was heard from the patient until several months later when an attorney contacted the hospital administration. The attorney asked whether the hospital was interested in settling a claim on behalf of the patient for physical injury sustained when a broken ammonium capsule was left on her stretcher and came into prolonged contact with the skin of her thigh. The capsule had caused a burn that took over 6 weeks to heal and required multiple visits to her physician. After investigating the situation, the hospital offered the patient a minimal settlement to cover her medical expenses.

The case was placed as an adverse outcome in the physician's peer review file.

Analysis

The fact that the patient was intoxicated and that the ammonium capsule created damage slowly over a period of many hours meant that the patient herself was unable to let the staff know that there was a problem while she was still in the emergency department. This cautionary tale illustrates the point that whenever we use a device, be it a needle or a substance such as ammonium that can cause a chemical burn, we run the risk of injuring someone if the item is not safely disposed of.

Teaching Points

1. Do not become complacent about leaving needles and other devices that may cause harm on a patient's stretcher.

2. The same holds true for causing harm to other emergency department staff members. The fewer the people who come into contact with contaminated, sharp, or caustic material, the better. Many emergency departments, for example, have a wise policy in which the physicians dispose of their own sharps after procedures such as laceration repairs.

Case 84
Led by the Nose

The daughter of a 76-year-old woman found her mother sitting on the couch, rubbing her left shoulder. She said that she had fallen. The bruises on her forehead and both arms and legs had not been there a few days before. Her mother could give no details about the event— whether she had fainted or stumbled. There were dirty dishes in the kitchen and a broken flowerpot on the floor. The television set was on but turned to a blank channel.

The daughter drove the patient directly to the emergency department for evaluation and related to the emergency physician a list of general concerns about her mother's recent health. Three months ago the patient had driven several hundred miles by herself to visit a relative, took no medication, and rarely saw the doctor. For the past several weeks, however, she had been forgetful and less concerned about her appearance, and her balance seemed poor.

The emergency physician was fairly sure that he knew what the problem was. On first entering the room he had noticed a faint but unmistakable odor of ethyl alcohol in the air. The patient had been drinking. The problem was looking more and more like "closet alcoholism" complicated by family denial. He had seen a similar case two days ago in an elderly man who abused Listerine.

While examining the patient, the emergency physician asked how much she drank. He had to repeat the question several times, not only because she seemed not to comprehend, but also because there was a boisterous patient on the other side of the curtain. She admitted to an occasional glass of brandy. He asked about how many bottles of brandy she might drink in a week. She stated that a bottle of peach brandy given to her for Christmas 5 years ago was still half full. The emergency physician then questioned the daughter, trying to get an idea of how much she knew or suspected. The daughter was a blank; in fact, the physician later said, she had seemed angry at his line of questioning.

The patient's vital signs were normal, and the brief general exam was remarkable primarily for a variety of bruises. Again, the physician sensed the faint odor of alcohol. He ordered an x-ray of the shoulder, which was negative. Although he was tempted to undertake a work-up, the day was busy and the patient was stable. He decided to let the patient's primary physician unravel the problem and discharged her with instructions to follow up as soon as possible.

The daughter called for an appointment, but the first available slot was 2 weeks later. Meanwhile, several days after the first emergency department visit, the patient fell again and injured her knee. The daughter, who had been spending nights at her mother's house to care for her, took her to a different emergency department. A second emergency physician listened to the daughter's story and performed a thorough neurologic exam. He discovered a marked pronator drift and several other abnormalities. He ordered a CT of the head and discovered a large brain tumor.

The daughter wrote the first hospital to complain about how far off base, not to mention insulting, the emergency doctor had been and that she would never come there again.

As it turned out, the director of the emergency department had been the double-cover physician that day, and it was not difficult to piece together what happened. The loud patient in the next cubicle had been intoxicated and was the source of the odor of alcohol.

Analysis

Snap judgments and immediate impressions are a necessary part of the practice of emergency medicine. Without them the physician could not take immediate action in acute life-threatening situations. But snap judgments clearly have a negative side, as this case illustrates. The physician walks into the patient's cubicle, smells alcohol, hears the story, and thinks that he has uncovered another closet alcoholic. End of search. He forces everything else to fall into line behind his initial mistaken notion.

First impressions—no matter how neatly they may seem to resolve a quandary—must be tested. They must not hamper the process of *worst case scenario thinking*. The wise physician is comfortable with uncertainty until all available evidence is on the scales.

The (unseasoned) physician's decision to let the primary care physician figure out why the patient had been deteriorating physically and mentally over the past weeks was not in the least prudent. Why had she fallen? He ignored the possibility of cardiac disease as well as a wide variety of metabolic, neurologic, and even hematologic abnormalities. The differential diagnosis, for that matter, also contained the possibility of elder abuse.

The patient should have been approached as a potential case of syncope in the setting of recent physiologic and cognitive deterioration. She deserved a careful exam and general studies and was a candidate for admission.

Teaching Points

1. If you suspect a patient of occult alcoholism, attempt at least to confirm the possibility with laboratory testing.

2. Elderly patients with unexplained falls are victims of syncope until proved otherwise.

3. Allow worst case scenario thinking to counterbalance the tendency to make leaps of judgment.

4. Exhalations from a single drunk patient can permeate entire segments of emergency departments. Do not let them pollute your judgment.

Case 85
The Artful Disposition

A 29-year-old woman presented with a history of flu-like symptoms for several days, including marked myalgias, joint discomfort, fever, headache, and nausea. She had no sore throat, cough, vomiting, or diarrhea. She was previously healthy and taking no medication. The emergency physician discovered no unusual findings. Her vital signs were normal except for a temperature of 100.1° F. Because of the benign exam, he ordered no laboratory tests and discharged the patient with a diagnosis of "viral illness." He did not give specific follow-up instructions.

The patient's myaglias and arthralgias progressed dramatically, however, and 6 days later she sought care at a primary physician's office, where a number of tests were performed. She was subsequently diagnosed with rheumatoid arthritis. At the suggestion of the primary physician, she called the hospital to complain of the misdiagnosis and to contest the bill.

Analysis

It may appear that the emergency physician discharged his primary responsibility toward the patient, and that he should not have been expected to pick up this uncommon diagnosis based on her initial presentation. But he could have averted this complaint. The diagnosis of "viral syndrome" is a great catch-all in modern medicine—the equivalent of "humoral imbalance" from a Galenic physician of a thousand years ago. In this particular patient, the combination of nonspecific myalgias and arthralgias, accompanied by malaise and a low-grade temperature for several days, is at best unusual for most viral illnesses, in which patients will manifest some respiratory or gastrointestinal symptoms as well. Therefore, a more accurate diagnosis would have been idiopathic febrile illness with myalgias and joint pain. One begins to think of autoimmune diseases or such atypical infectious conditions such as Lyme disease.

This is not to say that the physician should have made the correct diagnosis in the emergency department. In general, the emergency department is not the best place to search for such problems. But the patient warranted two considerations not provided by the emergency physician. The first is a diagnosis other than "viral illness." An honest statement such as "I don't know what's going on with you" would not have left the patient with the impression that she was misdiagnosed. Secondly, the emergency physician, given the fact that he was dealing with a clinical mystery that might turn out to be an uncommon condition, should have made more definite follow-up plans for the patient. As it turns out, she did not have a primary doctor of her own, and the physician's discharge instructions did not even mention follow-up.

Teaching Points

1. In the setting of the emergency department, where many cases must be discharged without definitive diagnoses, well-planned follow-up instructions are essential.

2. Do not be afraid to say, "I don't know."

3. Good follow-up plans are more important in mysterious cases.

Case 86
You Won't Want to Miss It

A young couple brought their previously healthy 8-week-old infant to the emergency department around midnight because he had "stopped breathing." He was their first child. The event occurred about 10 PM. The mother had been at work, and the father was babysitting. He stated that the child seemed to stop breathing for about a minute. He denied seeing any seizure activity. The child had been fine all day before the event.

The emergency physician found no signs of respiratory distress. The child was afebrile, and his pulse rate was 125 beats/min. His oxygen saturation was 100% on room air. The physician wrote on the chart that the child seemed "somewhat lethargic, might be sleeping." The exam was benign, but the emergency physician documented the presence of what looked like two bruises or either side of the child's chin.

The physician ordered a chest x-ray, which was negative. During the study the child become active and alert. During an hour-long stay, the child showed no respiratory distress. The emergency physician discharged him with instructions to see the pediatrician if any problems arose.

The mother, however, did not like the way the child looked or acted in the morning. He would not feed. She took him to the emergency department of a children's hospital in a nearby city, where a CT revealed intracranial bleeding. In addition, they discovered that the child had several bruises on his back and retinal and vitreous hemorrhages. The infant was admitted and discharged 2 weeks later into foster care.

The father was taken into custody and confessed to having shaken and thrown his son. The state health department cited the first emergency physician for poor documentation and failure to take due steps to evaluate and protect the child.

Analysis

Definite red flags were missed by the emergency physician: the odd nature of the event, the lethargy, the unexplained bruising, even the youthfulness of the parents and the fact the mother had not been at home. If the emergency physician had asked, he would have discovered that she was working because the father was unemployed. None of these elements by themselves indicated child abuse, but the sum total definitely merited great suspicion. "Shaken baby syndrome" can have widely varying and subtle presentations, but the child's lethargy, along with the episode of respiratory distress and the unexplained bruises, should have triggered an aggressive evaluation.

Any physician who has had to sit in a room with a child and its parents under similar circumstance recognizes the urge to believe that child abuse did not occur. Even to consider the possibility opens a Pandora's box of emotions, all of which are unpleasant—and some are almost unthinkable. A common first reaction on the part of inexperienced physicians is denial.

Obviously, the problem is real. The emergency physician must include child abuse in the differential diagnosis for any infant or child who presents with unusual symptoms or trauma. Only by walking into the room with this thought in mind is the physician likely to avoid missing subtle cases. Usually, child abuse can be excluded quite easily on circumstantial grounds without the family even being aware that it was a concern. Only when factors warrant further suspicion is the concern brought to the surface and steps taken to investigate.

If child abuse is a remote concern, but the physician believes it does not warrant further concern, he or she should document the possibility. If you make a practice of documenting concern about child abuse, you are more likely to think of it in the first place.

Teaching Points

1. Keep child abuse in the differential diagnosis for any infant or child who presents with changes in level of consciousness, respiratory episodes, unexplained bruising, inconsistent histories, or any degree of trauma.

2. If the clinical circumstances lead you away from the diagnosis of child abuse, make sure that you document why.

3. Have a low threshold for ordering CT scans of the head and for doing a good fundoscopic exam to check for retinal hemorrhages in any child at risk for shaken baby syndrome.

Case 87
Not a Happy Ending

A previously healthy 3-year-old boy was brought into the emergency department on Sunday because for the past several days he had been vomiting occasionally and acting generally irritable. His vital signs were perfectly normal, and his exam was benign. There were no signs of trauma or infection. His activity level seemed normal for his age, and he drank liquids in the emergency department without problems. The emergency physician did not believe that lab tests were indicated and discharged the patient with a diagnosis of possible "resolving viral syndrome."

The patient returned two nights later and was seen by a different emergency physician. His parents reported continued vomiting and episodes of seeming to fall asleep while playing. They were clearly anxious. Vital signs and exam were again unremarkable. The boy was afebrile and had no meningeal signs. The physician ordered a complete blood count and urinalysis and observed the patient for two hours. During this period the child fell asleep but aroused normally with stimuli. After the lab tests returned normal, the emergency physician called the patient's pediatrician to discuss the case. No further work-up seemed in order that night, and plans were made for the child to be seen in the office on the next afternoon.

On the following morning the patient was brought back to the emergency department by ambulance after a sudden spell of profound unresponsiveness during which one pupil transiently dilated. On arrival, however, the child was alert, and the vital signs and exam were once again unremarkable. The emergency physician suspected the presence of atypical seizure activity and ordered a CT. While waiting for the CT to be performed, the patient had a several-minute episode of limpness during which his left pupil dilated. The CT scan was expedited and revealed a mass lesion.

The patient was transferred quickly to a tertiary care center, where an astrocytoma was diagnosed. The patient underwent neurosurgery, but his prognosis was not good.

The patient's mother sent a letter of complaint to the hospital administration because the problem had not been diagnosed during the first two emergency department visits.

Analysis

Brain tumors are the most common solid tumors of childhood, with a peak incidence at age 5–10 years. As illustrated by this case, the early findings of central nervous sytem (CNS) tumors can be quite nonspecific. Signs and symptoms may include vomiting, lethargy, seizures, ataxia, and decrease in previously acquired motor skills. Preverbal children, of course, do not complain of headaches.

The first two emergency physicians, by any measure, did a reasonable job—although neither had considered the possibility of a CNS tumor. Most emergency physicians encounter only a few pediatric brain tumors during their clinical careers. The key to diagnosis involves keeping the disease in mind when dealing with any child with unexplained vomiting, ataxia, lethargic spells, or events that may represent typical or atypical seizure activity. Pediatricians include a CT scan in the work-up of such patients, and so must the emergency physician.

Teaching Points

1. Keep the diagnosis of brain tumor in mind when evaluating an afebrile child with unexplained vomiting, ataxia, lethargic spells, changes in cognitive or motor behavior patterns, or events that may represent typical or atypical seizure activity.

2. Order a CT scan, and involve the follow-up physician in the diagnosis of any patient who fits this picture.

Case 88
Help from Any Quarter

A 35-year-old man presented to the emergency department with complaints of intermittent left flank pain for 3 days. The pain was mild to moderate and had never become severe. He had no nausea but reported that his urine looked bloody from time to time. According to the emergency physician's brief note, he was a previously healthy man with no major medical problems and no history of kidney stones. Other than recent weight loss and fatigue, his review of systems was normal. He was taking no medications. His vital signs were normal. The emergency physician documented that he was a tired-looking, slender man who was in no acute distress. The exam was completely unremarkable. The emergency physician ordered a urinalysis and a kidney-ureter-bladder x-ray study—both of which were totally normal, although the radiologist noted the presence of considerable stool in the colon. No blood was found in the urine. Based on these findings and the lack of pain consistent with renal colic, the emergency physician did not pursue the diagnosis of kidney stone.

The physician told the patient he was not sure exactly what the problem was and recommended a bottle of magnesium citrate and a visit with the family physician after the weekend if the symptoms persisted.

On the next day, a Saturday, the man's wife called the emergency department and asked to speak with the supervisor. The clerk handed the phone to the medical director, who happened to be the physician on duty. The man's wife was extremely upset that nothing more had been done for her husband. His pain seemed a little better after the magnesium citrate took effect, but he still looked extremely sick. How could the physician say that he was just constipated? She wanted to file a complaint. The director suggested that she bring her husband for a reevaluation.

Several hours later, the man returned and was seen first by the nurse practitioner student on rotation. After spending over half an hour interviewing and examining the man, the student presented the case to the director. They examined him together, after which they discussed the best course of action. Although the vital signs were normal, the director had been impressed by how ill and fatigued the man appeared. There was periorbital puffiness and thinning of the skin. In fact, the director wrote in his note, the man looked at first glance like a renal dialysis patient. He told the student that they were likely to discover something like nephrotic syndrome or autoimmune glomerulonephritis. While deciding which lab tests to order, the student suggested a thyroid-stimulating hormone (TSH) test because of a family history of thyroid disease. The director humored the student but told her that there was essentially no chance of its being useful. The patient did not fit any picture of thyroid disease of which he was personally aware.

The lab tests returned. Again the urine was normal, with no trace of protein or blood. The completed blood count showed only slight anemia. The serum chemistries, including blood urea nitrogen and creatinine, were normal.

The TSH, however, was extremely high at 154 μU/ml (normal 0.85–2.32). The patient was profoundly hypothyroid. He was admitted and given high doses of levothyroxine. Within several days of treatment, his physician reported that the man looked like he had just "crawled out of a cave." The consulting endocrinologist said that if the diagnosis had been missed for several more weeks, the patient may have entered an irreversible myxedema state.

Analysis

Myxedema is an uncommon, life-threatening presentation of severe hypothyroidism characterized by physiologic decompensation. It is usually a geriatric disease. The signs of myxedema include decreased mental status, hypothermia, bradycardia, hypoventilation, periorbital edema, nonpitting edema ("peau d'orange"), delayed deep tendon reflexes, hypoglycemia, and hyponatremia. In extreme cases, the patient may become comatose. Here was a young man headed in that direction.

Simple uncomplicated hypothyroidism, on the other hand, is quite common. Primary hypothyroidism may have idiopathic or autoimmune causes or be related to iodine deficiency or postablation states. Less commonly, hypothyrodism may be caused by pituitary or hypothalamic disease. Medications, including amiodarone and lithium, also can cause thyroid hormone deficiency. Hypothyoridism is more common in women, and its onset is usually insidious, with such signs and symptoms as fatigue, hoarseness, weight gain, cold intolerance, periorbital puffiness, depression, peripheral neuropathy, delayed relaxation of ankle jerks, menstrual irregularities, loss of outer third of eyebrow, constipation, rough and dry skin, joint pains, muscle cramps, and bradycardia.

The director, in retrospect, said that the patient's thyroid had seemed "a little prominent" on examination, but he had not factored hypothyroidism into his differential diagnosis. The patient simply did not fit the picture. Other clues, however, should have triggered consideration of this possibility—fatigue, periorbital puffiness, and dry skin. Both physicians would have been justified in considering hypothyroidism based on the constellation of signs and symptoms and their chronicity.

This case illustrates how clinicians focus on a single, dramatic and familiar symptom—in this case, flank pain—and fail to consider the general picture. Everyone looked initially for a renal cause. But what was the actual cause of the flank pain? It was probably caused by intestinal colic secondary to hypothyroid-induced constipation.

We should be humbled by the thought that the patient might have been discharged a second time, still undiagnosed, if it were not for an astute nurse practitioner student.

Teaching Points

1. Thyroid disease should be suspected in any patient with nonspecific constitutional symptoms that last for more than 1 week, especially when routine lab tests have yielded no significant clues.

2. In dealing with a puzzling patient such as this, time spent on a review of systems and family history can yield important benefits.

3. Listen to the thoughts of students and trainees. They are closer to the land of zebras and more likely to act "by the textbook."

Case 89
A Lame Situation

The day after moving from one apartment to another, a previously healthy 22-year-old woman came to the emergency department complaining of feeling "achy" all over her body, especially in the legs, back, and arms. The patient was taking no medications other than birth control pills and denied similar symptoms in the past. She was afebrile. Her blood pressure was 120/72 mm Hg, and her pulse rate was 96 beats/min.

The emergency physician recorded that the review of systems was negative except for recent urinary frequency. On exam the patient was alert and oriented. The head, eye, ear, nose, and throat exam was normal, the chest was clear, and the abdomen was soft and nontender. He did not mention any muscle tenderness. He asked the nurse to give the patient an intramuscular dose of ketorolac, 60 mg, and to collect a specimen for urinalysis.

The urinalysis showed 10–15 white blood cells and 5–10 epithelial cells, and the dipstick was heme-positive, although no red blood cells were seen on the microscopic exam. The physician discharged the young woman with prescriptions for sulfamethoxazole-trimethoprim and propoxyphene/acetaminophen. His discharge impression was "lame muscles and UTI." The nurse's final note stated that the patient left "guarding with ambulation."

On peer-review the next day, another emergency physician flagged this patient as a potential missed case of rhabdomyolysis. She attempted to call the patient back for follow-up without success. A law enforcement officer went to her apartment and was told that the patient had gone to a different emergency department because the pain was worsening and her urine had turned dark. A subsequent call to the second hospital revealed that the patient had been admitted for intravenous hydration and observation. Further conversation with the attending physician at the second facility revealed that the patient had been using cocaine on the day of her move and that creatine kinase (CK) peaked at over 20,000 IU/L. She developed transient renal failure but subsequently did well.

Analysis

Rhabdomyolysis results from the breakdown of muscle tissue due to various causes, including crush injuries, overexertion, heat-related illness, and infections. Most emergency physicians probably see rhabdomyolysis most frequently in patients who present after intoxication with alcohol and various drugs, especially cocaine.[1] Rhabdomyolysis usually is accompanied by acute myalgias and muscle weakness, but not always. In advanced cases, patients may present with dark urine. Some patients have swollen, tender muscles, either diffuse or localized, but this finding is often absent. Serum CK is the most sensitive diagnostic test; a 5-fold increase establishes the diagnosis. Myoglobin also is elevated, but it is less sensitive than CK for making the diagnosis. Other nonspecific lab findings include hyperkalemia and abnormal calcium and phosphorus levels.

As many as 75% of patients also have myoglobinuria. Myoglobin cross-reacts with the urine dipstick assay for hemoglobin. A characteristic finding in rhabomyolysis, therefore, is a heme-positive dipstick without red cells on microscopic exam. This sign, however, is not sufficiently sensitive enough to be a universal screening test for rhabomyolysis.

The most common complication of rhabdomyolysis is acute myoglobinuric renal failure, which usually can be treated conservatively with fluids and alkylinization of the urine but mandates a search for rhabmyolysis in any patient at risk.

The young woman's complaint of diffuse myalgias in the setting of physical exertion[2] (even without the cocaine history that later surfaced) should have triggered thoughts of rhabmyolysis and the ordering of a CK test.

The emergency physician ordered a urinalysis because the patient complained of frequency, and in so doing missed a second, serendipitous opportunity to make the diagnosis when the urine was heme-positive without red blood cells.

The diagnosis of "lame muscles" was more than a little lame, as was the diagnosis of urinary tract infection, because the presence of epithelial cells indicated that the specimen was not a clean catch; therefore, the pyuria was of questionable diagnostic value.

Teaching Points

1. Think of rhabdomyolysis in any patient with myalgias, with or without muscle tenderness, especially after crush injuries, exertion, or heat-related illnesses and in the setting of drug or alcohol abuse.

2. CK is the best test to screen for rhabdomyolysis, and a 5-fold increase makes the diagnosis.

3. Three-fourths of patients with rhabdomyolysis demonstrate myoglobin in the urine, characterized by a heme-positive dipstick and no red blood cells on microscopic examination of the urine.

4. Patients with rhabdomyolysis are at risk for acute renal failure and require admission.

References

1. Counselman FL, et al: Creatine phosphokinase elevation in patients presenting to the emergency department with cocaine-related complaints. Am J Emerg Med 15:221, 1997
2. Sinert R, et al: Exercise-induced rhabdomyolysis. Ann Emerg Med 23:1301, 1994

Case 90
Taking a Back Seat

A surgeon sent a 70-year-old man with chronic obstructive pulmonary disease (COPD) to the radiology department for a chest x-ray for follow-up of a suspected lung mass. After the film, the patient began to have marked dyspnea. While walking back to the surgeon's office next door, he collapsed and was brought into the emergency department in extreme respiratory distress with marked hypotension. The emergency physician immediately intubated him. The surgeon rushed to the emergency department and began to perform the resuscitation, ordering the emergency physician—a recent emergency medicine residency graduate—to get blood gases and start a second intravenous line. The emergency physician did as he was asked.

The resuscitation continued for half an hour without success, and the patient died. A chest x-ray had not been ordered. An autopsy was not performed, and the cause of death noted on the death certificate by the surgeon was respiratory and cardiac arrest.

On routine code review the following day, the physician reviewer asked why tension pneumothorax had not been considered.

Analysis

It is well known that patients with COPD are at risk for spontaneous pneumothorax because of the presence of pulmonary blebs that can rupture under certain conditions. There are two iatrogenic conditions under which these blebs can easily rupture: (1) when the patient is ventilated too rapidly though an endotracheal tube and the lungs become overinflated and (2) when the patient takes a deep breath and holds it during the performance of a chest x-ray. During the length of his or her career, every emergency physician is likely to see at least one patient with COPD who suffers a spontaneous pneumothorax after a routine chest x-ray. If luck holds, that patient is still viable on reaching the emergency department, and the condition will be recog-

The end result system Codman (1900s)

Anesthesia study Commission (1935)

→ choose
Polumis
apt

→ email Joan
Brunch
9/8/06 & 9/13/06
yes pick up

nized as something other than a COPD exacerbation. If it is not, the risk of creating a tension pneumothorax is great.

We will never know if this patient had a tension pneumothorax. The emergency physician said that once the surgeon "pushed him out of the way," he became procedure-focused. The surgeon later stated that the possibility of a tension pneumothorax was "highly unlikely on clinical grounds."

In any case, we can only look to the future and state unequivocally that emergency physicians must keep tension pneumothorax high on the differential list when a patient with COPD has respiratory decompensation—especially after a chest x-ray.

Fortunately, the vast majority of consultants and admitting physicians are not interested in taking cases away from the emergency physician or inserting themselves uninvited into the responsibility chain. But the emergency physician must remember that if another physician tries to take control without a valid reason, along with documentation to verify it, the emergency physician will not escape liability for any adverse outcome. As long as the emergency physician is in the room or in any way involved in the case, he or she must continue to exercise clinical judgment.

Teaching Points

1. Always suspect a tension pneumothorax in patients with COPD who are rapidly deteriorating.

2. Never relinquish your clinical judgment when confronted by a senior clinician who wants to take over the case. The primary responsibility belongs to the emergency physician as long as the patient is in the department.

3. There is a real risk of creating a spontaneous pneumothorax when ventilating patients with COPD or asthma through the mechanism of "air trapping" if not enough time is allowed for the prolonged expiratory phase.

Case 91
The Last Nine Yards

A 64-year-old woman came to the emergency department complaining of a toothache. A left lower molar had been bothering her for the past week. She had no history of the same pain and was in generally excellent health. She had not seen a doctor since her general practitioner had died more than a decade ago, and she currently had no relationship with a primary care provider. The emergency physician examined her. The left second mandibular molar was exquisitely tender to percussion with a tongue blade, and tenderness and fullness were present in the adjacent buccal gutter, although no swelling was externally visible.

The emergency physician was preparing to write a prescription for penicillin when he looked over the vital signs in the triage note and saw that the nurse had mentioned "irregular pulse." He confirmed this finding: the rate was normal, but the rhythm was not. He decided to do a quick general exam and get more history. He went though a brief review of systems, quickly uncovering recent weight loss, malaise, and polydypsia and polyuria. He ordered an EKG and routine blood work. The cardiac rhythm turned out to be multifocal atrial tachycardia. The labs tests revealed a hemoglobin of 8.8 mg/dl and a random blood glucose of 290 mg/dl.

The emergency physician contacted the on-call internist's office, confirmed an appointment for the following day, instructed the patient to watch her intake of sweets in the meantime, and discharged her.

Later the next day the nurse manager of the emergency department came to the medical director with a concern from emergency nursing about the patient. Why had the emergency physician kept a patient with toothache in the emergency department for over 3 hours and ordered all sorts of extra lab tests?

Analysis

Clearly there are times during the course of an evaluation for a given clinical problem when the emergency physician has no ethical or professional choice but to follow-up on incidentally discovered abnormal findings that point toward additional problems. This was such a situation. Despite the fact the patient had no cardiac symptoms, the irregular pulse was abnormal and worrisome in her age range. She needed a cardiogram. The history of weight loss, malaise, and polydipsia/polyuria also demanded some sort of a laboratory investigation.

The nurse manager agreed to the cardiogram, but why the lab tests? Why not have them done the next day by her primary care physician? Why tie up a room in the emergency department and back up patient flow?

Emergency physicians are faced every day—like all modern medical practitioners—with conundrums over resource utilization. To some extent, it is a *damned if you do, and damned if you don't* situation. In the above case, the emergency physician may have argued himself out of doing lab tests based on the fact that no obvious acute illness needed immediate discovery. Simply informing the patient of his concern and warning her of the necessity to seek follow-up may have completely discharged his responsibility. On the other hand, the patient was a stoic woman who had no primary care physician and stated that she did not like going to doctors: "Just do something for my tooth, please, and I'll go see a dentist." She may well have failed to make the follow-up appointment with the internist until she became far sicker. And that, in fact, is exactly what the emergency physician, fresh out of his residency training, stated that he feared would occur. For this reason he said he went the extra nine yards. By clearly proving that she had glucose intolerance, he was able to convince her of the need for follow-up and, just as importantly, to get her firmly wedged into the busy primary care physician's schedule at an earlier date.

The physician showed good clinical judgment in the service of the patient's well-being. In the emergency department environment there are always conflicts between doing as much as we would like for patients and keeping the flow of patients as efficient as possible. Balancing these goals is one of the emergency physician's greatest challenges. Each emergency physician must exercise his or her best judgment in such situations. If there is a sound reason for pursuing an incidentally discovered sign or symptom, err in favor of the patient.

Teaching Points

1. Acute coronary syndromes sometimes present as jaw pain or toothaches. The patient's complaint may have been a sign of cardiac ischemia. The emergency physician was aware of this possibility, which was reflected in his documentation. He stated that the patient's toothache was not associated with chest pain, was nonradiating and present continuously, and gradually increased for three days. Furthermore, the physician mentioned her lack of cardiac risk factors.

2. Make it a firm habit to review the vital signs of all patients.

3. The test for pursuing an incidentally discovered finding is simple: If it will have a significant effect on the patient's well-being or help to identify the need for follow-up—go for it.

Index